Quality of Life Among Cancer Survivors

Tanya R. Fitzpatrick
Editor

Quality of Life Among Cancer Survivors

Challenges and Strategies for Oncology Professionals and Researchers

Springer

Editor
Tanya R. Fitzpatrick
Department of Social Work
Arizona State University
Westmount, QC, Canada

ISBN 978-3-030-09174-3 ISBN 978-3-319-75223-5 (eBook)
https://doi.org/10.1007/978-3-319-75223-5

Softcover re-print of the Hardcover 1st edition 2018

Printed on acid-free paper

This Springer imprint is published by the registered company Springer International Publishing AG part of Springer Nature.
The registered company address is: Gewerbestrasse 11, 6330 Cham, Switzerland

Brief Summary

This book will provide specific information to health and oncology professionals who are preparing to or who already work and conduct research with cancer survivors both in hospital and community settings. From the perspective of several disciplines, cancer survivors facing different types of challenges will be explored. Social and health issues from a multidisciplinary approach will provide further meaning and insight into interventions that attempt to address the complex challenges of living with a chronic and sometimes fatal disease.

Tanya R. Fitzpatrick

Introduction

This book will provide specific information to oncology professionals and researchers who are preparing to or who already work and conduct research with cancer survivors both in hospital and community settings. From the perspective of several disciplines, cancer survivors facing different types of challenges will be explored to better understand and provide insight into useful strategies to assist these groups. Social and health issues from a multidisciplinary approach will highlight interventions that oncology professionals can use to address psychosocial and health-related issues among cancer survivors living with a chronic and sometimes fatal disease.

Frequently, a cancer "survivor" is defined as a person who has lived 5 years after diagnosis; however, the definition has been expanded to include people diagnosed from the onset of the disease until recovery or death and that can include many more years (Canadian Cancer Society, 2010). Although cancer survivors have an increasingly longer life span due to more advanced medical treatment and care, emotional and physical challenges and barriers to treatment are a constant reminder of the day-to-day struggle to survive. A good number of cancer survivors experience the fear of recurrence (Maheu, 2016), physical symptoms of pain and fatigue, cognitive and memory impairment, plus symptoms related to their particular type of cancer effecting their quality of life (Mititelu, Aruljothy & Fitzpatrick, 2016).

Despite recent advances and management of the disease including earlier detection, newer treatments, rehabilitation and the management of symptoms, the quality of life of surviving patients with cancer must focus on the psychological, physical, social, and spiritual well-being. However, growth of the cancer patient population does not parallel the supply of oncology physicians and other healthcare professionals to meet the unmet needs that will increase as patients progress through " the continuum of diagnosis, treatment, survival, and possible relapse" (Chasen, Hollingshead, Conter, & Bhargava, 2017, p. 151). Meterissian (2017) reports that the healthcare system is "slow to recognize the need to treat the human being, not only the disease" (P. A6). Emphasis should now be placed not only on the increasing cost of healthcare and treating illness and injuries that is needed, but also on the importance of " whole person care" (Meterissian, 2017), and the "care plan process."

This includes an interdisciplinary approach and integrated care between the physician, the oncology team, the patient and his/her family members, followed by a rehabilitation plan to "promote a return to functional capacity and self-management" (Chasen et al., 2017, p. 151).

This book will highlight the approaches of several different disciplines and their perspectives on case management and interventions that attempt to promote emotional and physical health, the provision of information, access to resources, and attention to quality of life. Although considerable research has addressed different therapeutic interventions and quality of life among cancer survivors (Fitzpatrick, 2016; Fitzpatrick & Farone, 2011; Edgar, 2016; Fitch, 2009; Fitzpatrick & Remmer, 2011), the field of cancer survivorship is relatively new and remains an emerging field (Jezer-Morton, 2015; Mayo, 2001; Maheu, 2016). Mayo (2015) believes that one of the reasons is that no one profession has taken it on. Regardless, the field of oncology has emerged as including many disciplines collaborating together to address common goals similar to the field of gerontology. Fields such as medicine, social work, nursing, rehabilitation, psychology, psychiatry, genetics, dentistry, medical ethics, and social ethics will be explored as they relate to various oncology issues.

This book distinguishes itself from previous literature, specifically from an earlier book entitled *Treating Vulnerable Populations of Cancer Survivors* (Fitzpatrick, 2016), because it will include new perspectives from disciplines such as bioethics, genetics, medicine, dentistry, nursing, social work, and psychology.

The first chapter by Dr. Fitzpatrick briefly explores several theoretical perspectives in an attempt to clarify the relationship between quality of life and therapeutic interventions adapted to address the challenges of cancer survivors, for example, play and leisure activities, and physical fitness activities. Chapter 2 also by Dr. Fitzpatrick focuses on cognitive health and quality of life among older cancer survivors introducing the concept of "Play" along with exploring the benefits of leisure activities as interventions promoting better cognitive health especially among those undergoing chemotherapy. This is followed in Chap. 3 by Yasi Xiao focusing primarily on older Chinese cancer survivors and issues of acculturation and health-related quality of life. Clinical and ethical issues are addressed in Chap. 4 by Robert Orr outlining the identification, analysis, and resolution of ethical dilemmas that arise in the care of individual cancer patients. In Chap. 5, Janice Berlinger and Megan Fleischut examine genetic mutations in cancer susceptibility genes among family members with cancer. They present two case analyses and describe treatment options focusing on the BRCA2 gene and the mutation of the RBI gene. Dr. Feras Al Halabi, a dentist treating cancer patients, presents literature in Chap. 6 on the quality of life among patients with tongue cancer in which speech and swallowing are greatly effected. Chapter 7 by Dr. Leimanis and Ms. Zuiderveen focuses on issues of intensive care and rehabilitation for hospitalized children with cancer. Chapters 8 and 9 by Michelle Le and Veronique Huot provide a comprehensive literature review on post-traumatic stress disorder and quality of life addressing family and sibling relationships among pediatric cancer survivors.

In Chap. 10, Fatima Boulmalf addresses young adult survivors of childhood cancer and provides an intensive review of several theoretical perspectives in order to further examine the relationship between post-traumatic stress disorder and quality of life. For example, the concept of cognitive vulnerability, the terror management theory, the anxiety disruption buffer theory, and the social causation and social erosion hypotheses are discussed in this chapter. Dr. Laizner continues in Chap. 11 by focusing on family functioning and presents therapeutic interventions addressing family members with cancer. Following this, in Chap. 12, Dr. Bushfield focuses on family caregivers and the Hospice team when cancer returns among survivors. The final chapter, Chap. 13, by Jack Phelan discusses cancer services from a personal cancer experience and suggests survival challenges and strategies for healthcare providers to address some of the barriers and ongoing supports for cancer survivors.

This book also provides further insight into issues of cognitive health, hospice and palliative care, ethnicity and acculturation, health-related quality of life, gender differences among family caregivers, and complex sibling relationships. A variety of therapeutic interventions will also be discussed such as play therapy and leisure activity, social support groups, physical fitness, and brain fitness activities in an attempt to address the needs of cancer survivors and the ways that community service providers can respond to them.

References

Canadian Cancer Society. (2010). *Breast Cancer Statistics*. Retrieved from http://www.cancer.ca.

Chaput, G. (2015). In Rachel Lou (2015). Surviving cancer: The struggle continues for treatment. March 5/2015. (On-line Production).

Chasen, M., Hollingshead, S., Conter, H., & Bhargava, R. (2017). Quality of life for patients surviving cancer: Are we moving ahead? *Current Oncology, 24,* 151–152.

Edgar, L. (2016). Providing psychosocial distress screening, coping resources and self-care to newly diagnosed cancer survivors in a canadian small town setting. In T.R. Fitzpatrick, (Ed.), *Treating vulnerable populations of cancer survivors: A biopsychosocial approach* (pp. 7–22). 10.1007/978-3-319-32364-0_2.

Fitch, M. I. (2009). Supportive care framework: Theoretical underpinnings. *Supportive Care Framework: A foundation for Person-Centered Care.*(Pappin Communications).

Fitzpatrick, T. R., & Remmer, J. (2011). Needs, expectations and attendance among participants of a cancer wellness centre in Montreal, Quebec. *J Cancer Survivors, 5*(3), 235–246. doi: 10.1007/s11764-011-0176-8

Fitzpatrick, T. R. (2016). *Treating vulnerable populations of cancer survivors: A biopsychosocial approach.* (Ed. T. R. Fitzpatrick). Switzerland: Springer International Publications.

Jezer-Morton, K. (2015). Cancer survivorship: A new field? In *McGill Medicine: FOCUS,* Fall 2015.

Maheu, C., Lebel, S., Courbasson, C., … & Sidani, S. (2016). Protocol of a randomized controlled trial of the fear of recurrence therapy (FORT) intervention for women with breast or gynecological cancer. *BMC Cancer.*

Mayo, N. (2015). In Jezer-Morton, K. (2015). Cancer survivorship: A new field? *McGill Medicine Focus, Fall,* (pp. 14–15).

Mayo, N., Scott, S. C., Shen, N., Hanley, J., Goldberg, M. S., & MacDonald, N. (2001). Waiting time for breast cancer surgery in Quebec. *CMAJ, 164*(8), 1133–1138.
Meterissian, S. (2017). The importance of whole person care. In *The Montreal Gazette, Thursday, Oct. 12, p. A6).*
Mititelu, R., Aruljothy, A., & Fitzpatrick, T. R. (2016). Physical activity, locus of control, and fear of recurrence among cancer survivors from a community-based cancer support program. In T. R. Fitzpatrick (Ed.) (2016). *Treating vulnerable populations of cancer survivors: A biopsychosocial approach.* Switzerland: Springer International Publications.

Contents

Contributors

Janice L. Berliner works as a senior genetic counselor at Memorial Sloan Kettering Cancer Center. She earned her Masters of Science in Human Genetics and Genetic Counseling from the University of Michigan and is licensed by the state of New Jersey. With over 28 years of experience in prenatal, pediatric, and mostly cancer genetics, Janice enjoys assessing her patients' genetic predispositions to cancer, providing risk assessment, education, and counseling. Her main research interest involves risk assessment and genetic counseling for hereditary breast and ovarian cancer.

Fatima Boulmalf is a second-year medical student at McGill University Faculty of Medicine. She graduated from the Pure and Applied Sciences (Honors) program at Vanier College (Montreal) on the Dean's List and has since been working on projects pertaining to high-value care and resource stewardship training in medicine. She is co-president of the High-Value Care Club and a Choosing Wisely Canada student leader. She is passionate about civic engagement and advocacy, and is the newly appointed VP Campaigns Québec of the McGill Government Affairs and Advocacy Committee (GAAC).

Suzanne Young Bushfield began her 40-year career as a social worker in healthcare, working in oncology, hospice, and behavioral health. She served on the faculties of Arizona State University, New Mexico State University, Lewis Clark State College, and the University of North Dakota. Dr. Bushfield's research has focused on issues which have an impact on women's lives throughout the life span, including breast cancer, and end-of-life caregiving. She ended her career as an Accreditation Director for the Council of Social Work Education and as Chief Accreditation Operations Officer for the Association for the Accreditation of Human Research Protection Programs.

Tanya R. Fitzpatrick obtained her Ph.D. from Boston College Graduate School of Social Work and is Professor Emerita from Arizona State University in Phoenix, Arizona (Dept. of Social Work) with a background in nursing, oncology, and gerontology. Prior to this, she served on the faculties at Boston College and the University of St. Josephs in West Hartford, CT. More recently, she was the Director of Research and a Consultant at Hope & Cope at the Jewish General Hospital in Montreal, Quebec (2009–2013). She continues to mentor first- and second-year McGill Medical students on research focusing on cancer survivors and health-related outcomes. Besides editing a book on ethnic elders and a more recent book on cancer survivors, she has received grants, and published numerous articles and book chapters in scientific journals.

Megan Harlan Fleischut is Manager, Clinical Genetics Service at Memorial Sloan Kettering Cancer Center. She is a board-certified genetic counselor with over 14 years experience in clinical cancer genetics. She received her Masters of Science in Genetic Counseling from the University of North Carolina at Greensboro while training at the hospitals affiliated with Duke University, the University of North Carolina at Chapel Hill, and Wake Forest University. Megan joined MSKCC's Clinical Genetics Service in 2006. As the Service's Manager, she collaborates with a team of 15 genetic counselors, 5 physicians, and several administrative leaders and support members. Megan's primary research interest is on retinoblastoma survivors.

Feras Al Halabi completed an Honors Bachelor of Science in Immunology from McGill University in Montreal and a Doctor of Dental Medicine at McGill University in 2013. He pursued postgraduate internship training in oral and maxillofacial surgery at the Montreal General Hospital. Following this, he began working on studies related to oral cancer interventions and quality of life outcomes associated with these interventions. He is involved in undergraduate teaching at McGill University's Faculty of Dentistry. He is an active member of the Association des chirurgiens dentistes du Québec (ACDQ), the Canadian Dental Association (CDA), and American Dental Association (ADA).

Véronique Huot is a third-year medical student in the Class of 2019 at McGill University, Faculty of Medicine, Montreal, Quebec. She graduated with distinction from the University of Calgary in 2014 with a Bachelor of Kinesiology. Her interest in oncology comes from her three years volunteering at the Thrive Centre, an innovative fitness facility aiming to empower and improve quality of life of people affected by cancer, which is located at the University of Calgary. Her major research interests focus on physical activity, oncology, and pediatrics.

Andréa Maria Laizner is a Nursing Practice Consultant at the McGill University Health Centre, Associate Researcher in the MUHC Research Institute's Cancer Program, and Assistant Professor at McGill University Ingram School of Nursing. Her research focuses on comfort and symptom management in diverse populations across the life span. She is involved in health services research related to best practice guidelines and knowledge translation to provide patient- and family-centered care. Recently, she received funding from the Rossy Cancer Network to adapt the Canadian Association of Psychosocial Oncology "Start the Talk" web-based information modules, which she co-authored in French.

Michelle Le completed her undergraduate degree at the University of Ottawa and is currently a third-year medical student at McGill University. Michelle has a great interest in research, specifically in oncology and immunology. Having experienced the impact of a loss due to cancer first hand, Michelle is a strong advocate for interdisciplinary care for cancer survivors. She looks forward to continuing her medical and research pursuits in hopes to improve knowledge translation in the field of oncology.

Mara L. Leimanis completed her Ph.D. at McGill University, Montreal, Canada, in 2008, and then spent postdoctoral research in Asia with Oxford University. She then completed several projects at McGill University and worked at the Jewish General Hospital in the Hope & Cope Cancer Support program. She currently holds an Adjunct Professor position with MSU and is a Research Scientist with Helen DeVos Children's Hospital in Grande Rapids Michigan. Her current research interests include biomarker development, precision medicine, oncology, and psychosocial issues for acutely ill pediatric intensive care patients.

Robert D. Orr practiced family medicine in rural Vermont for 20 years. An interest in medical ethics led him to postdoctoral studies at the Maclean Center for Medical Ethics at the University of Chicago. Since that training, he has held professorships at Loma Linda University (CA), Trinity International University (IL), the Graduate School of Union University (NY), and the University of Vermont College of Medicine. He has lectured widely and contributed to the literature scores of books, chapters, case reports, and articles, with a primary focus on end-of-life care and clinical ethics consultation.

Jack Phelan has been in the CYC field for 50 years and has enjoyed it immensely. He is a faculty member at MacEwan University in Edmonton, Alberta, Canada, where he teaches in the Child and Youth Care degree program. Jack has recently published a book on child and youth care work and he will soon publish another on CYC supervision. Jack is a regular contributor to CYC-OnLine on the cyc-net website and is involved with doing workshops and presentations both in Canada and internationally.

Yasi Xiao is a fourth-year medical student at McGill University, Montreal, Quebec. Born in China, She immigrated to Canada from China with her mother at the age of 10. She began volunteering at the Chinese Family Service of Greater Montreal in High School, working mostly as an interpreter for unilingual Chinese elderly during their medical appointments. Yasi has a wide range of interest in medicine and her passion is to improve the experience of immigrants in the Canadian healthcare system.

Sandra K. Zuiderveen is a Clinical Database Specialist at VPS Site Coordinator for Helen DeVos Children's Hospital/Spectrum Health System Grand Rapids, MI. After earning her BSN at Calvin College, she spent 6 years working at

Children's Hospital of Michigan in Detroit. In the summer of 1998, she has worked for Spectrum Health ever since, and has worked as the data collector for VPS and finally Site Coordinator for VPS in 2008. She enjoys the details of data collection and sometimes digging for the most accurate data. Multiple projects and research studies have utilized VPS data throughout the years with several more planned for the near future. As a result, she has managed to co-author several peer-reviewed articles.

Chapter 1
Theoretical Perspectives

Tanya R. Fitzpatrick

This chapter will discuss various theoretical and conceptual models to provide further insight into the relationship between therapeutic interventions, quality of life, and social and health issues among cancer survivors. Information from these perspectives should provide further understanding and useful guidelines for oncology professionals and family caregivers. These theories have a common thread in that they attempt to explain the process of cancer survivorship and quality of life in which good adjustment in later life is positively associated with participation in various activities (Fitzpatrick, 1995; Zarit, 1980). With the longer period of survival along with the rapid increase in new technological, detection, and medical interventions, the goal of not only prolonging life but attempting to address the ongoing challenges that cancer survivors and their family caregivers face becomes more important.

Cancer Survivorship and Quality of Life

The concept of *quality of life* has emerged as an important addition to understanding therapeutic interventions and cancer survivorship because loss of physical capacity and lifestyle is experienced by many individuals who are diagnosed with cancer (Fitzpatrick, Edgar, & Holcroft, 2012). Quality of life is a broad multidimensional construct which includes the participants' self-appraisal of mood, coping resources, and self-esteem (Haes, 2004), plus emotional, social, sexual, cognitive, and physical functioning (Yanez, Thompson, & Stanton, 2011).

T. R. Fitzpatrick (✉)
Department of Social Work, Arizona State University, Westmount, QC, Canada
e-mail: Tanya.fitzpatrick@asu.edu

T. R. Fitzpatrick (ed.), *Quality of Life Among Cancer Survivors*,
https://doi.org/10.1007/978-3-319-75223-5_1

Addressing the relationship between therapeutic interventions and quality of life among cancer survivors from a multidisciplinary perspective, several theories and models may assist in furthering to understand this relationship.

Stress and the Coping Mechanism

Following the diagnosis of most forms of cancer, many individuals experience difficulty in managing their daily life and adjusting to the physical health changes that are occurring. Reactions may include distress or extreme stress, anxiety and depression, and thoughts of avoidance, plus fear and confusion as to their future well-being (Leimanis & Fitzpatrick, 2014). However, the stress and suffering that is attributed during the cancer survivorship journey may be understood through the stress and coping mechanism and the individual's ability to coping with their illness (Barroihet Diez, Foriaz, & Garrido Landivar, 2005). Coping can be defined as the ways and means that an individual uses to adjust and adapt to the cancer (Folkman & Greer, 2000). Yet it can also be said that coping may not always be effective in attempting to control overwhelming amounts of distress because of one's living arrangements and other demographic factors such as age, gender, marital status, education, race, and religion which can present barriers to effective coping and/or accessing services (Fitzpatrick, 2016).

Activity Theory

Activity theory (Maddox, 1988, 2001) also known as the implicit theory of aging, normal theory of aging, and lay theory of aging proposes that successful aging occurs when older adults stay active and participate in social activities. The activity theory perspective (Fitzpatrick, 1995, 2010; Littman, Tang, & Rossing, 2010; Maddox, 2001; Speck, Courneya, Masse, Duval, & Schmitz, 2010; Zarit, 1980) may assist in clarifying the relationship between various forms of activities and interventions and quality of life among cancer survivors of all ages. Participation in physical and/or social activities has been positively associated with reducing stress and having a beneficial effect on well-being among older adults (Fitzpatrick, 1995). Furthermore, physical activities such as yoga, aerobics, strength-based exercises, and cardiovascular training are said to protect against cognitive decline in cancer survivors when memory impairment or confusion may occur following chemotherapy (Fitzpatrick et al., 2012).

The *direct effect model* and the *stress-buffering hypothesis* as conceptualized by Wheaton (1985) propose that any form of social support or a coping resource may

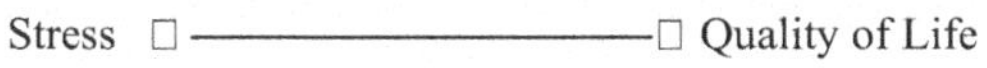

Fig. 1.1 The direct effect model

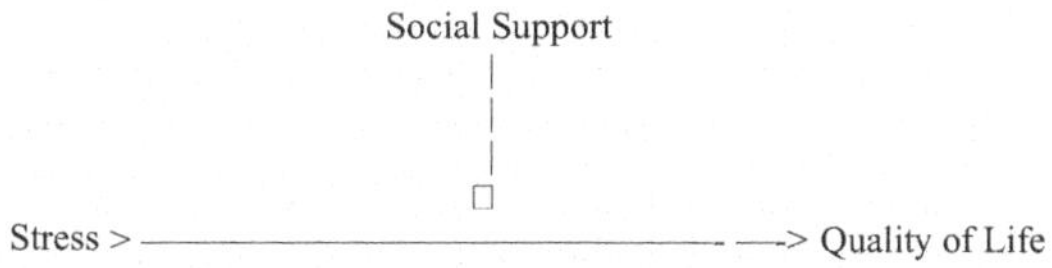

Fig. 1.2 The stress-buffering hypothesis (Wheaton, 1985)

serve as a moderator or buffer to mediate the negative effects of stress or any other negative outcome. Social support in the form of various interventions directly acts on the original stress to alleviate or make less severe the negative outcome.

Specifically, the *direct effect model* would suggest that stress from a cancer diagnosis would act directly on quality of life, thus decreasing or having a negative effect on the individuals' sense of well-being and quality of life. Therefore, in the direct effect model, stress acts negatively and directly on quality of life (Fig. 1.1 represents the direct effect model).

The *stress-buffering model* as proposed by Wheaton (1985) incorporates both the concept of social support and the stress coping model.

Social Support and the Stress-Buffering Model

Social support may be provided in the form of emotional or instrumental support received from family members, friends, and the community or supports provided from professionals. Many forms of social supports that provide opportunities for social interaction, such as recreational activities including various social and physical activities (Fitzpatrick, 1995), leisure activities (Fitzpatrick & Farone, 2011), group support interventions, and/or support and care provided by family members, can have an ameliorating effect on stress and/or other negative physical and emotional health outcomes (Cohen & Wills, 1985; Farone, Fitzpatrick, & Tran, 2005). Considerable research suggests that the presence of social support can serve to reduce psychological distress (Berkman, Glass, Brissette, & Seeman, 2000; Cohen & Wills, 1985; Fitzpatrick, Gitelson, Andereck, & Mesbur, 2005; Fitzpatrick, McCabe, Gitelson, & Andereck, 2005) and certainly cancer survivors face stress-related decisions and challenges once they have received a diagnosis of cancer. Therefore, various forms of social supports are seen to provide beneficial effects on quality of life, especially for cancer survivors (Fitzpatrick & Farone, 2011; Leimanis & Fitzpatrick, 2014) (Fig. 1.2 represents the stress-buffering hypothesis in which social support acts directly on the relationship between stress and quality of life).

Summary

Exploring the relationship between different forms of therapeutic interventions found in group and community programs may serve to buffer or make less severe the negative effects of stress or depression. This gains importance as evidence suggests that the use of various forms of supportive activities will have a beneficial effect on mental and physical health outcomes among cancer survivors (Leimanis & Fitzpatrick, 2014). Therefore, stress can be modified or reduced by the addition of social supports or coping resources to providing a beneficial effect on quality of life (Fitzpatrick & Farone, 2011).

The theories and models described above are not exhaustive, but they allow us to place these theories within the context of useful interventions. This is important for oncologists and service care professionals working and providing care for cancer survivors. The knowledge from this book should also encourage students focusing their practice and research in oncology to view each individual cancer patient or survivor with a new sense of understanding leading to address more adequately the physical and mental health needs of this vulnerable group of individuals. Therefore, the quality of life of cancer survivors and their family members depends on in-home and community-based supports that address not only their medical needs but highlight their emotional and psychosocial needs as well (Smith-Osbourne & Felderhoff, 2014).

References

Barroilhet Diez, S., Foriaz, M. J., & Garrido Landivar, E. (2005). Concepts, theories and psychosocial factors in cancer adaptation. *Actas Españolas de Psiquiatría*, *33*, 390–397.

Berkman, L. F., Glass, T., Brissette, I., & Seeman, T. E. (2000). From social integration to health: Durkheim in the new millennium. *Social Science & Medicine*, *51*(1982), 843–857. https://doi.org/10.1016/S0277-9536(00)00065-4

Cohen, S., & Wills, T. A. (1985). Stress, social support and the buffering hypothesis. *Psychological Bulletin*, *98*, 310–357.

Farone, D. W., Fitzpatrick, T. R., & Tran, T. V. (2005). Use of Senior Centers as a stress-coping strategy among Latino elders. *The Journal of Gerontological Social Work*, *46*, 65–83.

Fitzpatrick, T. R. (1995). Stress and well-being among the elderly: The effect of recreational services. *Journal of Applied Social Sciences*, *19*, 95–105.

Fitzpatrick, T. R. (2010). Brain fitness activities and health among female Senior Center participants in Montreal, Quebec. *Journal of Activities, Adaptation and Aging*, *34*, 30–47.

Fitzpatrick, T. R. (2016). *Treating vulnerable populations of cancer survivors: A biopsychosocial approach* (pp. 1–2). AG Switzerland: Springer International Publishing.

Fitzpatrick, T. R., Edgar, L., & Holcroft, C. (2012). Assessing the relationship between physical fitness activities, cognitive health and quality of life among older breast cancer survivors. *Journal of Psychosocial Oncology*, *30*, 556–572.

Fitzpatrick, T. R., & Farone, D. W. (2011). Leisure, household activities and health among Mexican American elders with cancer. *Journal of Psychosocial Oncology*, *29*, 199–214.

Fitzpatrick, T. R., Gitelson, K., Andereck, K., & Mesbur, E. S. (2005). Social support and health among a Senior Center population in Southern, Ontario, Canada. *Social Work and Health Care*, *40*, 15–37.

Fitzpatrick, T. R., McCabe, J., Gitelson, R., & Andereck, K. (2005). Factors effecting perceived social and health benefits among senior center participants. *Activities, Adaptation and Aging*, *30*, 23–45.
Folkman, S., & Greer, S. (2000). Promoting psychosocial wee-being in the face of serious illness: When theory, research and practice inform each other. *Psycho-Oncology*, *9*, 11–19.
Haes, J. C. M. (2004). The distinction between affect and cognition in the quality of life of cancer patients-sensitivity and stability. *Quality of Life Research*, *1*, 315–322. Activity theory (aging) – Wikipedia https://en.wikipedia.org/wiki/Activity_theory_(aging)
Leimanis, M., & Fitzpatrick, T. R. (2014). Physical activities and distress among participants of a cancer wellness centre: A community-based pilot study. *International Journal of Physical Medicine and Rehabilitation*, *2*, 1–8. https://doi.org/10.4172/2329-9096.10000193
Littman, A. J., Tang, M.-T., & Rossing, M. A. (2010). Longitudinal study of recreational physical activity in breast cancer survivors. *Journal of Cancer Survivorship*, *4*, 119–127.
Maddox, G. L. (1988). *Aging and well-being. The 1987 Boettner Lecture*. Bryn, Mawr, PA: Boettner Research Institute.
Maddox, G. L. (2001). *The encyclopedia of aging: A comprehensive resource for gerontology and geriatrics* (3rd ed.). New York, NY: Springer Pub.
Smith-Osbourne, A., & Felderhoff, B. (2014). Veterans' information care givers in the sandwich generation: A systematic review toward a resilience model. *Journal of Gerontological Social Work*, *57*, 556–573.
Speck, R. M., Courneya, K. S., Masse, L. C., Duval, S., & Schmitz, K. H. (2010). An update of controlled physical activity trials in cancer survivors: A systematic review and meta-analysis. *Journal of Cancer Survivorship*, *4*, 87–100.
Wheaton, B. (1985). Models for the stress-buffering functions of coping resources. *Journal of Health and Social Behavior*, *26*, 352–364.
Yanez, B., Thompson, E. H., & Stanton, A. L. (2011). Quality of life among Latina breast cancer patients: A systematic review of the literature. *Journal of Cancer Survivorship*, *5*(2), 191–207. https://doi.org/10.1007/s11764-011-0171-0. Epub 2011 Jan 28.
Zarit, S. H. (1980). *Aging and mental disorders*. New York, NY: The Free Press.

Chapter 2
Play, Leisure Activities, Cognitive Health, and Quality of Life Among Older Cancer Survivors

Tanya R. Fitzpatrick

Introduction

The purpose of this chapter is to explore the relationship between play, leisure activities, cognitive health, and quality of life among older cancer survivors. Older cancer survivors in particular face not only the detrimental effects of a cancer diagnosis but also age-related chronic diseases and/or physical limitations. In addition, for those who have undergone chemotherapy, cognitive impairment known as "chemo-brain or chemo-fog" (Bury, 2017; Fitch, Armstrong, & Tsang, 2008) has been associated with cognitive changes on quality of life among elderly cancer survivors (Fitzpatrick, Edgar, & Holcroft, 2012).

Past studies have established a strong relationship between the benefits of leisure and household activities on several physical and mental health outcomes among older Mexican American cancer survivors (Fitzpatrick & Farone, 2011) and between both older and younger Latino cancer survivors (Fitzpatrick, 2016). However, few studies have examined the relationship between what is termed "play" and what is meant by "leisure activities" which may serve to benefit or contribute to maintain cognitive health during the survivorship phase. New research has shown the cognitive benefits of play for older as well as younger adults (Brown, 2009; Hoehn, 2014; Lamberton, 2016). As older adults live longer, brain diseases may become more prevalent (McCabe, 2017). However, all cancer survivors face numerous challenges following the diagnosis, and their quality of life can be greatly impacted. It is therefore necessary to identify useful interventions that will maintain and even promote better cognitive health among cancer survivors. The aims of this chapter will be to explore various forms of play and leisure activities and their differences and similarities and how they impact cognitive health and quality of life. This chapter will focus on the following:

T. R. Fitzpatrick (✉)
Department of Social Work, Arizona State University, Westmount, QC, Canada
e-mail: Tanya.fitzpatrick@asu.edu

T. R. Fitzpatrick (ed.), *Quality of Life Among Cancer Survivors*,
https://doi.org/10.1007/978-3-319-75223-5_2

1. Review of the literature on cognitive health, quality of life, and cancer
2. Theoretical perspectives
3. Therapeutic interventions
4. A case example of a man suffering from prostate cancer and chemo-related symptoms
5. Implications for clinical practice and future research

Cancer, Chemotherapy, and Cognitive Health

Cognitive heath, defined by the National Institute of Health (NIH), is the conservation of cognitive structures that enables adults to maintain social connectedness, a sense of purpose, and functional autonomy and to cope with arising life stressors (Rogers, Larkey, & Keller, 2009). A study by Beard, Fetterman, Wu, and Bryant (2009) found that those with a history of cancer may experience long-term effects on mental and physical health conditions as well as on neurocognitive functioning. Furthermore, those undergoing chemotherapy may experience what is known as "chemo-brain or chemo-fog" (Fitch et al., 2008; Fitzpatrick et al., 2012). Many patients have reported that their memory, thinking, perception, and ability to concentrate have been altered following chemotherapy and this in turn has affected their quality of life. In addition, many report that cognitive difficulties remain even after a decade following treatment (Evans & Eschiti, 2009). For elderly patients in particular, chemotherapy-related impairment may go underdiagnosed as it can often be confused with depression or other chronic illnesses (Fitzpatrick et al., 2012: Raffa et al., 2006).

Confusion and memory impairment as a result of chemotherapy can increase stress by producing negative physical and emotional outcomes. Additionally, stress from living with a cancer diagnosis can "degrade" brain function especially when referring to memory and cognition (Pellis, Pellis, & Himmler, 2014, p. 73). Pellis et al.'s (2014) studies on adult animals found that stress levels decreased after engaging in play, suggesting that play may serve as a means to reduce stress in adults and protect the brain from confusion and deterioration. The prefrontal cortex of the brain is responsible for behaviors such as emotional response, impulse control, and mood regulation; however, positive and playful interactions are needed to keep the brain functioning at peak performance (Pellis et al., 2014). Implications from this research suggest that there are cognitive benefits from "play" for adults. It is therefore important to highlight cognitive health and its relationship to quality of life by studying various forms of interventions involving physical activity and social involvement.

Theoretical Perspectives and Conceptual Models

Many of the theories that were described in Chap. 1 can apply to all cancer survivors and older adults but also those suffering from cognitive impairment as a result of chemotherapy either recent or in the past. However, in this chapter, several additional perspectives will be described. The *social cognitive theory* as proposed by Hoffman, Lent, and Raque-Bogdan (2013), although not specifically addressing cognitive impairment from chemotherapy, can be applied as a form of intervention for those cancer survivors suffering from memory or confusion. The social cognitive model of restorative well-being is a framework to understand those coping with early-stage adult cancer (i.e., stages I and II) and "optimizing post-treatment adjustment" (Hoffman et al., 2013, p. 242). The model therefore emphasizes strengths and positive adjustment outcomes. These authors also focus on survivorship research addressing cancer-related coping strategies such as efficacy beliefs, personality traits, and environmental supports, "which have been linked to positive adjustment outcomes and thus may inform psychosocial interventions" (Hoffman et al., 2013, p. 242). This research is grounded in a theoretical base to assist oncology workers, psychologists, social worker, and nurses in providing services to elderly cancer survivors.

Activity theory as proposed by Fitzpatrick (1995), Maddox (1988, 2001), Courneya (2003), and Zarit (1980) is useful in understanding the relationship between activities such as play and/or leisure activities and cognitive health among older cancer survivors. Cognitive health can be defined in the context of this chapter as confusion and memory loss resulting from those undergoing chemotherapy or other forms of treatment that may result in impaired thinking (Ahles & Saykin, 2001, 2002; Fitzpatrick et al., 2012). The study by Fitzpatrick et al. (2012) found that participation in physical activities had a positive effect on cognitive health and quality of life among breast cancer survivors who were undergoing chemotherapy.

Social Support Theory

In the event of a life-threatening diagnosis of cancer, the individual is faced with an increasing amount of stress associated with uncertainty and fear about their future. Social support is a mechanism that can reduce stress "by resources provided by others of the stressful event thus allowing the individual a means of adjusting or recovering from a difficult situation" (Fitzpatrick, Kressin, Bossé, Spiro III, & Greene, 2001; p. 220). Reinforcement and feedback from others helps to validate and recognize the difficulty of the situation and may also help to maintain the individual's self-esteem and self-worth (Krause, 1986). According to Wheaton (1985), a person who is experiencing a stressful life event such as cancer yet has a strong social support network from family and friends or in the community, the negative effect of stress can be reduced by the positive nature of a social support resource. Social support can act as a mediator or can moderate the detrimental effects of the stressful situation and make it less severe.

Similarly, Bernard, Zysnarska, and Adamek (2010) define two types of social support: emotional and practical. *Emotional support* received from friends, family, and health professionals allows the individual to cope in a better manner with their own fears and anxiety by discussing their concerns with others who are usually understanding and sympathetic and may offer needed acceptance and validation. *Practical support* aims at the exchange and provision of information and advice that can bring about a better understanding of their condition, life situation, and problems by serving to provide exchange and feedback of information about their disease and the services and community supports that can assist. Social support, by participating in social events and leisure activities, can also serve as a mediator to ward off and make less severe cognitive impairment as a result of chemotherapy (Fitzpatrick et al., 2012).

The Stress and Coping Mechanism

When one is confronted with a cancer diagnosis, fear and confusion may result as to the uncertainty of their present and future health status and from the fact that there is no escape from the diagnosis. The stress and coping mechanism is the process and ability of the individual to adapt during a lengthy survivorship journey, which can be a life-threatening disease. Coping is defined as "the specific thoughts and behaviors that a person uses in his/her efforts to adapt to the cancer" (Folkman & Greer, 2000, p. 11). Barroilhet Diez et al. (2005) state that the stress and coping mechanism explains the influence of coping to cancer including sociocultural, psychological, and medical factors. Edgar (2010, 2016) presents an introduction to basic coping strategies to further empower cancer patients and their families. In a book on coping strategies, Edgar (2010) includes information on what is "good coping" and tools for coping such as exercise, remembering how you successfully coped in the past, dealing with a changed healthcare system, deep breathing, and mindful meditation. In addition, the process of coping and adapting to a cancer diagnosis may also be understood from the perspective of the stress-buffering model.

The Stress-Buffering Hypothesis and Model

Play and leisure activities may be seen as a form of social support and serve to reduce or modify the negative effects of memory or confusion associated with cognitive impairment among cancer survivors. Wheaton (1985) conceptualized a pathway beginning with an environmental stressor such as cancer. The individual therefore may experience stress as a result of exposure to the changes in their health and life status. The challenge of coping with a life-threatening disease may lead to deleterious physical and emotional symptoms. Effective coping can reduce or eliminate the harmful effects (Edgar, 2016). Coping resources may be internal or external that can serve to buffer the negative effects of stress (Wheaton, 1985). The model is designed to assess whether a higher distress level is found among cancer survivors who participate in play and/or leisure activities and may in turn be associated with less cognitive difficulties. The following will demonstrate the stress-buffering models such as the *direct effect model*, the *mediating effect model*, and the *moderating effect model* of the coping resource.

The *direct effect model* posits that stress may act directly on the stressful situation to increase distress or cognitive impairment. (See Fig. 2.1 for the direct effect of stress.)

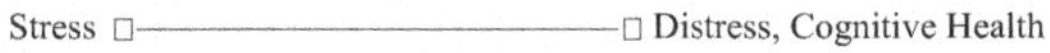

Fig. 2.1 Direct effect of stress

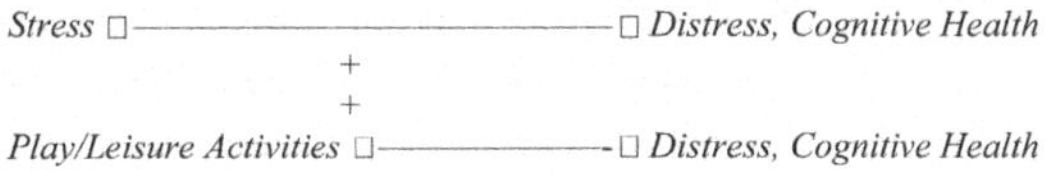

Fig. 2.2 The mediating effect of play or leisure activities

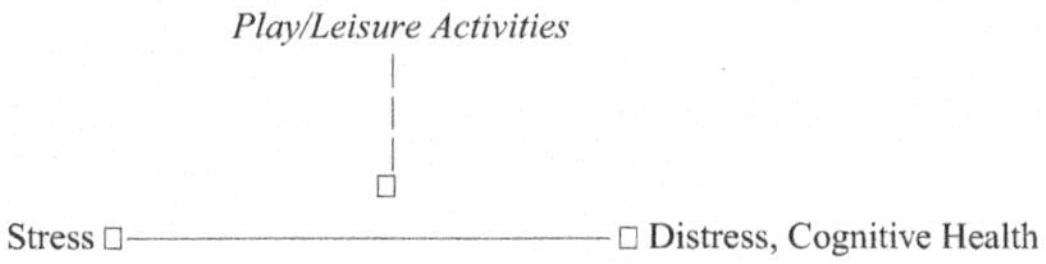

Fig. 2.3 The moderating effect (interaction effect) of play/leisure activities

The use of play and leisure activities is seen as a coping resource. Therefore, the *mediating effect model* tests the direct effect of stress *on* the distress of cognitive impairment and, therefore, adds the coping resource of play or leisure activities directly on the distress which is said to mediate the effects of stress on cognitive difficulties and make it less severe (see Fig. 2.2).

Finally, the coping resource (play or leisure activity) could have a *moderating and interaction* effect specific to exposure of the stress. Therefore, the coping or social support resource acts to reduce the impact of the stressor, rather than to directly reduce the stress. This model would test the interaction effect between stress and cognitive impairment by the addition of play or leisure activities. Note that play or leisure activities act directly on the relationship *between* stress and the distress of cognitive impairment and serve to moderate the effects and make it less severe (Farone, Fitzpatrick, & Tran, 2005; Wheaton, 1985) (See Fig. 2.3).

In summary, the theoretical and empirical work described in the above theories and models (social cognitive theory, activity theory, social support theory, stress and coping mechanism, and the stress-buffering models) examining the relationship between play and leisure activities on cognitive impairment attempts to clarify our understanding of this important relationship. One of the objectives of this chapter is also to discuss the similarities and differences between play and leisure activities and their role as an effective intervention in the maintenance of cognitive health and quality of life among older cancer survivors who are experiencing stress as a result of chemotherapy and cognitive impairment.

Therapeutic Interventions

Interventions designed to improve cognitive health and quality of life among cancer survivors are explored together with clinical implications for appropriate oncology and healthcare practice and future research.

State of Play

“Play” is a relatively new concept in adulthood as scientifically play has been seen as essential for childhood in the development of motor and social skills (Elkind, 2007) and has been shown to “stimulate the prefrontal cortex, the brain’s emotional center” (Lamberton, 2016, p. 74). The “state of play” as described by Lamberton (2016) is a cognitive health benefit serving as a stress reduction mechanism among children and also older adults. Lamberton defines “play” as “doing something that delivers enjoyment purely for its own sake” (Lamberton, 2016, pg. 74; Brown, 2009). Brown who founded the *National Institute for Play* in California further describes play as pleasurable and voluntary. Play activities can be also described as “purposeless” but can have long-term beneficial effects, not only for growing children but for older adults.

Activities associated with play can be as simple and noncomplicated as playing games with your grandchildren, reading a good novel, watching TV, shopping, or coloring in an adult coloring book, where the action itself is more important than the outcome. Even playing video games as “gamers” today includes all genders, races, and age groups. “Video games are truly ageless” (Jenkins, 2016, p. 38). Games are fun and provide a little respite from our busy day-to-day schedule, and they also serve as exercise for the brain (Jenkins, 2016). American Association for Retired People (AARP, 2017) offers games on aarp.org mostly for one player but is soon to include games that can be shared with family and friends.

Play activities do have similarities with activities associated with social and leisure pursuits. For example, recently, adult-specific play experiences are now offered at summer camps with opportunities to share a cabin with cabin mates and/or participate in arts and crafts and sing-alongs at campfires. Schulte (2014) in her research found that our imagination becomes alive when we permit ourselves to play using playful thinking. Schulte also states that play does not have to involve a time commitment or be expensive, but one can take at least 1/2 h out of a busy day, to do something enjoyable or something that we have enjoyed as a child. Older retired adults naturally have more time for play activities; however, adults who are working and raising a family may feel that they have little time for play, especially when it involves their own time (Schulte, 2014).

Leisure Activities

Cognitive functioning includes brain activities that are related to knowledge, memory, attention, and language to assess information. Aerobic exercise and physical activity are said to improve cognitive health across the life-span (Hillman, Erickson, & Kramer, 2008). A specific example is fitness training which is linked to improvement in various aspects of cognition. Regular exercise can do much to prevent cognitive dysfunction regardless of one’s age (Booth, Roberts, & Laye, 2012).

Leisure Activities, Cognitive Health, and Cancer

Leisure activities have been shown to reduce depression and contribute to positive self-reported physical health among elderly Mexican Americans with cancer (Fitzpatrick & Farone, 2011). Findings indicated that leisure participation, especially household activities, was significantly related to better self-reported health, less cutting down on activities and less depressive symptoms. Regular physical activities are part of leisure and recreational activities, work-related activities, and various forms of exercise programs (Eyler et al., 2002; He & Baker, 2004). Fitzpatrick et al. (2012) found that as physical fitness activities increased among older cancer survivors, cognitive health and quality of life improved for those on chemotherapy.

Leisure activities may include *social or solitary activities* (Fitzpatrick et al., 2001). Although some solitary activities are joined by others, solitary activities could include reading, walking alone, hobbies, watching TV, gardening work, or even household activities such as cleaning, washing, and shopping. These Activities could also be classified as "play" activities which were described above, whereas *social activities* usually involve different forms of physical and activities joined by others such as work-related activities, team sports, playing tennis, participating in a gym program or class, or caring for others, to name just a few. Fitzpatrick et al. (2001) found that leisure activities performed either alone or with others moderated the effects of stress on physical health but not mental health among bereaved elderly men. While these studies highlight the relationship between leisure activities and health outcomes among cancer survivors and bereaved elderly men, they do not address chemotherapy-related outcomes and cognitive dysfunction among cancer survivors. While activities in the form of physical fitness activities have been found to provide a beneficial effect on cognitive health and quality of life for those patients on chemotherapy, few studies have considered the benefits of "play" activities as they relate to cognitive impairment following chemotherapy. Regardless, older patients who have undergone chemotherapy, radiation, and/or surgery may experience loss of muscle strength, fatigue, or reduced cardiovascular capacity making it difficult to participate in leisure or even play activities during active treatment (Knobf, Thompson, Fennie, & Erdos, 2014). Additionally, cancer patients are sometimes left to deal with the negative effects of the very treatments that are prescribed to provide a cure (Park, 2016). As Park adds, these patients should be supported in the best way we can. It should also be understood that not all patients undergoing chemotherapy experience declines in cognitive functioning (Jansen, Miaskowski, Dodd, Dowling, & Kramer, 2005).

As we have seen from the literature, play activities have not been considered a unique concept apart from leisure because they can appear similar in many ways. Furthermore, some play and leisure activities involve others, yet both can be solitary as well. Regardless, both play a role as useful interventions to help maintain and provide some relief from cognitive difficulties following chemotherapy and other forms of treatment among cancer survivors. Nevertheless, other supportive interventions do play an important role in providing emotional and physical benefits along with play and leisure activities.

Physical Fitness Activities

Adamsen et al. (2003) and Fergusson and Gill (1991) report that regular physical activity provides a range of cognitive benefits to cancer survivors. The activity theory perspective (Fitzpatrick, 1995, 2012; Maddox, 1988; Zarit, 1980) is useful to understand the relationship between physical fitness activities and cognitive health especially in later life. Moderate participation in physical activities such as yoga, aerobics, strength-based exercises and cardiovascular training, and walking are said to protect against cognitive decline (Adamsen et al., 2003; Colcombe et al., 2006; Kamijo et al., 2009; Oken et al., 2006; Weuve et al., 2004).

Psychological Interventions

In combination with play, leisure, and physical fitness interventions, psychological interventions are also beneficial for cancer survivors such as support groups and psychotherapy (Leimanis & Fitzpatrick, 2014). Interventions from social support resources are imbedded in play and leisure activities and perhaps provide a double benefit, as the individual is not only receiving benefits from the actual participation but also receiving supportive feedback and companionship from others. As activity theorists suggest, the socialization aspect of activities involved in play, leisure, physical fitness, group therapy, education, and church-based interventions offers the cancer patient an opportunity to improve their health and quality of life especially for patients with cognitive difficulties (Fitzpatrick, 1995, 2016).

Social Support and Group Therapy

Social support can be defined as a mechanism that reduces the severity of stress by providing an opportunity for clarification through resources provided by others (Fitzpatrick et al., 2001). Social support groups offer a means for adjusting and coping during a stressful life situation by the providing reinforcement and feedback, thus helping to maintain the individuals' self-esteem and self-worth (Krause, 1986). Although there are support groups geared toward cancer survivors offered in some community cancer centers, leisure activities and physical activities also offer a group experience to help the individual socialize yet also come to terms with cognitive difficulties as a result of their illness and treatment. For example:

Mr. X is a 75-year-old man with a fairly recent diagnosis of prostate cancer and metastases to the bone. He has undergone chemotherapy over the past year and a half. Initially he complained of slight confusion and some memory loss. Before diagnosis, he was a very active family man, involved in his career and community activities. He continues these pursuits, time permitting in between his ongoing treatment. He has also begun a fitness and exercise group program in his community geared toward cancer survivors. He states that this program has helped to improve physical symptoms and also his memory. Naturally he has needed time to recover after each bout of chemotherapy which also impacted his sight and other physical symptoms such as fatigue, appetite, and mobility.

Group activities that offer social support which are hobbies, arts and crafts, team sports, exercising, community organizing, and especially learning a new language or learning to play a musical instrument are said to help maintain cognitive functioning during a stressful life experience such as cancer or Alzheimer's disease (McCabe, 2017). McCabe (2017) and colleagues from the Montreal Neurological Institute are helping to identify interventions that improve the quality of life for people with neurological disorders. *Senior centers*, although not all directed toward cancer survivors, offer an opportunity for group interventions and are said to help moderate stress-related distress among Latino elders with cancer (Farone et al., 2005). In addition, *focus groups* offer an intervention strategy proved to be beneficial to cancer survivors who participate in a group experience which can address a wide range of concerns and burdens that survivor face. They provide an opportunity to better understand and cope with the disease on a daily basis (Ceballos, Molina, Ibarra, Escareno, & Marchello, 2015).

Online support groups for cancer survivors are also an avenue for cancer survivors to explore, especially those who may be homebound. "Online support groups take place using a password-protected message board format (not live chat) and are led by professional oncology social workers who offer support and guidance. Groups are held for 15 weeks at a time, and group members must register to join. After completing the registration process (which can take up to 2-3 business days), members can participate by posting in the groups 24 h a day, 7 days a week." (Edlund, 2017, p.1).

Neurology and Oncology

Schagen, Klein, and Reijnrveld et al. (2014), as neurology oncologists, have explored cognitive functioning and current initiatives to assist patients with brain tumors during the course of cancer who develop cognitive problems resulting in functional dependence. Cognitive endpoints are defined as memory problems, attention, executive functioning, and speed processing, all of which affect quality of life. These authors discuss the precise mechanisms underlying treatment-related cognitive side effects as necessary to enable the identification of novel treatment strategies such as rehabilitation strategies and the important role of cooperative groups focusing on cognitive endpoints in clinical trials to assist in treating cognitive dysfunction. Castellino, Ullrich, Wjelen, and Lange (2014) review the epidemiology, pathophysiology, and assessment of cancer-related cognitive dysfunction among pediatric cancer survivors of brain tumors and leukemia who experience cognitive impairment months and even years after treatment. Preventive measures would include educational and pharmacological interventions to remediate established cognitive dysfunction following childhood cancer. "The increased years of life saved after childhood cancer warrants continued study toward the prevention and remediation of cancer-related cognitive dysfunction, using uniform assessments anchored in functional outcomes" (Castellino et al., 2014, p. 186).

Educational Activities to Maintain Brain Fitness

Cognitive impairment experienced by cancer patients can be severe and long-lasting, especially related to memory and attention (Pascal, 2015). Pascal states that problems in attention and memory can be controlled by either non-pharmacological, behavioral, pharmacological, and a combination of behavioral and pharmacological interventions, for example, by establishing daily routines, implementing reminders to aid memory, training in attention, increasing physical activity, cognitive behavioral therapy, improving nutrition and sleep, mental exercises and brain-plasticity-based cognitive training, and, if necessary, using specific medication, all of which to improve quality of life for cancer patients and survivors (Pascal, 2015).

A study at Memorial Sloan-Kettering in New York City by Kasven-Gonzalez (2017), an occupational therapist, offers a variety of strategies to help boost memory, enhance problem-solving skills, and improve awareness and judgment for patients who are suffering from cognitive difficulties as a result of chemotherapy or other treatments. The main focus is on increasing physical activity at a gym or at home to help combat fatigue, weight gain and bone loss, anxiety, and depression. (See brainhq.com for specific physical fitness exercises and activities.) An earlier study by Kasven-Gonzalez, Souverain, and Maile (2010) focusing on rehabilitation for palliative care patients to improve the quality of life found that occupational (OTs) and physiotherapy (PTs) interventions working in collaboration with patients could help set realistic and meaningful goals to achieve quality of life. Another research study explored the differences between physical activity and mental activity comparing which activity benefits the most for keeping the mind fit (Godman, 2015). Exercise alone protects the brain, and tests for mental activities showed brain shrinkage. Mental activities to improve memory would include crossword puzzles, reading, participating in groups and clubs, and learning a new language, but not passive engagement like watching TV. Active engagement seen in physical activities might include:

- Intensive computer work plus aerobics
- Intensive computer work plus light stretching and toning
- Watching educational DVDs plus aerobics
- Watching educational DVDs plus light stretching and toning

The researcher found no real differences between physical or mental activity groups on thinking tests, as all could exercise a particular brain function (Godman, 2015).

Summary of the Literature

Few studies have examined the relationship between "play" and "leisure" activities, cognitive health, and quality of life among cancer survivors. Cancer-related memory and attention limitations as a side effect from chemotherapy have been described *as chemo-brain or chemo-fog* (Fitch et al., 2008; Fitzpatrick et al., 2012). Patients have reported changes in their thinking, ability to concentrate and recall (Fitch et al., 2008). The purpose of this chapter was to explore the relationship between play and leisure activities as interventions for maintaining cognitive health and quality of life among cancer survivors. Besides describing in the literature review the benefits of "play" and "leisure" activities as related to cognitive health and quality of life, theoretical perspectives were examined as a means of assisting in understanding the relationship between these major concepts. Additionally, other supportive resources and interventions were included to demonstrate the benefits of physical activities, psychological interventions, social support groups, educational resources, neurology, and brain fitness exercises, all of which can be found in various play and leisure pursuits.

The theoretical and empirical work described in the theories and models of social cognitive theory, activity theory, social support theory, the stress and coping mechanism, and the stress-buffering models was helpful in guiding the work and linking the concepts, suggesting that participation in various forms of play and leisure activities is an important intervention in maintaining cognitive health and quality of life among older cancer survivors and those undergoing chemotherapy. Specifically, the concept of play was explored and can be seen as a useful activity that many individuals may participate in on a daily basis (Brown, 2009; Hoehn, 2014; Lamberton, 2016). Play can be recognized as a beneficial intervention both as a separate activity and also in combination with leisure activities. Additionally, if the individual is limited in physical mobility and is homebound as a result of recent chemotherapy, radiation, or surgery or is an elderly cancer patient with other chronic illnesses or dementia-related limitations, play activities can be found in the home environment as convenient and less physically demanding, for example, playing with grandchildren, reading, or doing puzzles. Recently, play activities are being included and developed in many playground spaces in the United States. The idea is based on the notion that we do not stop playing because we are old, suggesting that play and fun activities can continue throughout the life-span (Ianzito, 2017). Although the concept of play and leisure activities seems to involve similar forms of participation, leisure pursuits are not as spontaneous as play activities. Leisure activities are more structured and usually organized by community leaders and performed in community settings.

The activity theory suggests that participation in activities both solitary and social has a beneficial effect on mental and physical health among older adults (Fitzpatrick, 1995; Fitzpatrick et al., 2001; Maddox, 1988; Zarit, 1980) and on cognitive health and quality of life among cancer survivors (Fitzpatrick et al., 2012; Fitzpatrick & Farone, 2011). The findings from this chapter provide further support to investigations highlighting the benefits of exercise as a physical activity among cancer survivors (Kramer, Erickson, & Colombe, 2006; Littmen, Tang, & Rossing, 2010).

Based on the stress-buffering model, play and leisure activities can also serve as a social support intervention that can buffer and mediate the negative impact of stress from chemotherapy-related cognitive dysfunction (Fitzpatrick et al., 2012; Krause, 1986; Weave et al., 2004).

Implications for Clinical Practice and Research

The results of this chapter review have implications for clinical practice and future research to better inform patients and oncology professionals of the psychological and cognitive challenges resulting from chemotherapy and possibly other forms of treatment and the importance of participation in both play and leisure activities. As Fitzpatrick et al. (2012) point out, it is also necessary to evaluate the stage and type of disease and the form of treatment as this will affect the patient's ability to participate in various activities. Elderly cancer patients' circumstances may differ from those of younger adults or pediatric cancer survivors, and therefore it is necessary to match their limitations with realistic goals. Oncology professionals, physicians, nurses, social workers, OTs, PTs, and other staff should work collaboratively with exercise physiologists to ensure the proper balance of activities. In addition, oncology professionals addressing therapeutic interventions should promote the benefits of all forms of activities and especially activities which involve social interaction between other cancer survivors, family members, friends, and professional staff focusing on cognitive difficulties and quality of life.

Future research studies should investigate a broader community sample of individuals to gain further insight using personal interviews and reflections. A study by Fitzpatrick et al. (2012) did include 16 participants in which face-to-face interviews were conducted assessing the effects of physical fitness activities on cognitive health outcomes among older cancer survivors. Although the sample was small, the individual participants felt validated that their concerns were identified and ideas were discussed to address their cognitive needs. Further research should also assess different types of "play" activities. For example, the American Association for Retired People (AARP) in their recent monthly magazine includes an article that describes recreation as an endless recess in which playground-style equipment aimed at grown-ups is being installed in Marion Diehl Park in Charlotte, NC. This community has opened its second "intergenerational play space" in which many people are attracted to the social play as well as the physical play (Ianzito, 2017). Another program that was recently developed called "Java Memory Care" adapted from the "Java Music Club" was launched in 2011 is now in place in 600 senior homes across Canada and the United States (Jager, 2017). The Memory Care Program focuses on dementia where community volunteers team up with residents, both high- and low-functioning individuals, and attempts to build bonds and foster new and deeper relationship, which all in turn has a positive effect on well-being and quality of life (Jager, 2017). *Mindfulness-based cognitive therapy* (MBCT) is an example of a study that investigated the use of a MBCT group for older adults who were experiencing depression and anxiety (Foulk, Ingersoll-Dayton, Kavanagh, Robinson, & Kales, 2014). Findings revealed that group therapy and not pharmacological interventions were associated with positive changes. Mindfulness therapy has implications for further research among those cancer survivors who may be experiencing memory difficulties. In addition, the relationship between exercise and a healthy diet focusing on brain boosters or "brain waves" has recently been the study of current literature which identifies certain special foods that are positively related, such as black currents, broccoli, dandelion greens, kimchi (lactic acid bacteria), pumpkin seeds, sage, and turmeric, and, along with exercise, can stimulate the production of neurons and be "neuroprotective" (Zoomer: Vitality, 2017, p. 59). Additionally, besides food and exercise, learning a new language using an app on a computer can help combat cognitive aging. Furthermore, researchers from the University of Montreal highlight the significance of speaking two or more languages which may offset certain forms of dementia (Zoomer, 2017, October, p. 59). However, little research has investigated the effects these new programs have on cancer survivors and those with chemotherapy-related cognitive difficulties.

This investigation highlights the importance of play and leisure activities as interventions in the design and programming at community cancer support centers and also in institutional settings in an attempt to address the many challenges that cancer survivors face following chemotherapy and other forms of treatment. More sophisticated research in this area is warranted and could provide new insights for oncology researchers and healthcare professionals who are interested in facilitating groups or programs addressing cognitive health issues among cancer survivors. Such investments are likely to enhance the well-being and quality of life of all cancer survivors.

References

Adamsen, L., Midtgaard, J., Rorth, M., Borregaard, N., Anderson, C., … Knusten, L. (2003). Feasibility, physical capacity, and health benefits of a multidimensional exercise program for cancer patients undergoing chemotherapy. *Supportive Care in Cancer, 11*, 707–716.

Ahles, T. A., & Saykin, A. J. (2001). Cognitive effects of standard-dose chemotherapy in patients with cancer. *Cancer Investigation, 19*, 812–820.

Ahles, T. A., & Saykin, A. J. (2002). Breast cancer chemotherapy-related cognitive dysfunction. *Clinical Breast Cancer, 3*, S84–S90.

American Association of Retired People (AARP). (2017). *AARP The Magazine: Real Possibilities*. aarp.org.

Barriolhet Diez, S., Foriaz, M. J., & Garrido Landivar, E. (2005). Concepts, theories and psychosocial factors in cancer adaptation. *Actas Españolas de Psiquiatría, 33*, 390–397.

Beard, R. L., Fetterman, D. J., Wu, B., & Bryant, L. (2009). The two voices of Alzheimers: Attitudes towards brain health by diagnosed individuals and support persons. *The Gerontologist, 49*, 40–49.

Bernard, D., Zysnarska, M., & Adamek, R. (2010). Social support for cancer: Selected problems. *Reports of Practical Oncology & Radiotherapy, 15*(2), 47–50.

Booth, F. W., Roberts, C. K., & Laye, M. J. (2012). Lack of exercise is a major cause of chronic diseases. *Comprehensive Physiology, 2*, 1143–1211.

Brown, S. (2009). In S. Brown (Ed.), *Play: How it shapes the imagination and invigorates the soul*. NewYork, NY: Penguin Group Inc.

Bury, M. (2017). Review paper. Chemobrain in patients suffering from cancer based on the example of multiple myeloma. *Current Problems of Psychiatry, 18*(1), 62–69. https://doi.org/10.1515/cpp-2017-0006

Castellino, S. M., Ullrich, N. J., Wjelen, M. J., & Lange, B. J. (2014). Developing interventions for cancer-related cognitive dysfunction in childhood cancer survivors. *Journal of the National Cancer Institute, 106*(8), dju186. Published online 2014 Jul 30. https://doi.org/10.1093/jnci/dju186

Ceballos, R. M., Molina, Y., Ibarra, G., Escareno, M., & Marchello, N. (2015). Design, development, and feasibility of a Spanish-language cancer support group. *Support Care Cancer*. https://doi.org/10.1007/s00520-014-2549-9

Colcombe, S., Erickson, K., Scalf, P., Kim, J., Prakash, R., McAuley, E., … Kramer, A. (2006). Aerobic exercise training increases brain volume in aging humans. *The Journal of Gerontology: Medical Sciences, 61A*, 1166–1170.

Courneya, K. S. (2003). Exercise issues in older cancer survivors. *Medicine & Science in Sports & Exercise, 35*(11), 1846–1852.

Edgar, L. J. (2010). *Mastering the art of coping in good times and bad*. Ontario, Canada: Copelindaedgar.

Edgar, L. J. (2016). Providing psychosocial distress screening, coping resources and self-care to newly diagnosed cancer survivors in a Canadian small town setting. In T. R. Fitzpatrick (Ed.), *Treating vulnerable populations of cancer survivors: A biopsychosocial approach* (pp. 7–22). Springer Nature: Springer International Publishing AG Switzerland. https://doi.org/10.1007/978-3-319-32364-0_2

Edlund, C. (2017). On-line Support Groups. https://Cancercare.org

Elkind, D. (2007). *The power of play: Learning what comes naturally*. Cambridge, MA: De Capo Lifelong Books. http://dacapopress.com

Evans, K., & Eschiti, V. (2009). Cognitive effects of cancer treatment: Chemo brain explained. *Clinical Journal of Oncology Nursing, 13*, 661–666.

Eyler, A. E., Wilcox, S., Matson-Kauffman, D., Evenson, K. R., Sanderson, B., Thompson, J., … Rohm-Young, D. (2002). Correlates of physical activity among women from diverse racial/ethnic groups. *Journal of Women's Health & Gender-Based Medicine, 11*, 239–253.

Farone, D. W., Fitzpatrick, T. R., & Tran, T. V. (2005). Use of senior centers as a moderator of stress-related distress among Latino elders. *Journal of Gerontological Social Work, 46*, 65–83.

Fergusson, R. J., & Gull, A. (1991). Quality of life measurement for patients undergoing treatment for lung cancer. *Thorax, 46*, 671–675.

Fitch, M. I., Armstrong, J., & Tsang, S. (2008). Patient's experiences with cognitive changes after chemotherapy. *Canadian Oncology Nursing Journal, 18*, 180–192.

Fitzpatrick, T. R. (1995). Stress and well-being among the elderly: The effect of recreation-al services. *The Journal of Applied Social Sciences, 19*, 95–105.

Fitzpatrick, T. R. (2016). *Treating vulnerable populations of cancer survivors: A biopsychosocial approach* (pp. 1–2). AG Switzerland: Springer International Publishing.

Fitzpatrick, T. R., Edgar, L., & Holcroft, C. (2012). Assessing the relationship between physical fitness activities, cognitive health and quality of life among older breast cancer survivors. *Journal of Psychosocial Oncology, 30*, 556–572.

Fitzpatrick, T. R., & Farone, D. W. (2011). Leisure, household activities, and health among Mexican American elders with cancer. *Journal of Psychosocial Oncology, 29*(2), 199–214.

Fitzpatrick, T. R., Kressin, N. R., Bossé, R., Spiro, A., III, & Greene, E. (2001). Leisure activities and health among bereaved elderly men: The Normative Aging Study. *OMEGA: Journal of Death and Dying, 43*, 217–245.

Folkman, S., & Greer, S. (2000). Promoting psychosocial wellbeing in the face of serious illness: When theory, research and practice inform each other. *Psycho-Oncology, 9*, 11–19.

Foulk, M. A., Ingersoll-Dayton, B., Kavanagh, J., Robinson, E., & Kales, H. C. (2014). Mindfulness-based cognitive therapy with older adults: An exploratory study. *Journal of Gerontological Social Work, 57*, 498–520.

Goodman, H. (2015). Which is better for keeping the mind fit? Physical or mental activity? The Harvard Health Letter. *Harvard Medical School, Harvard Health Publications*. https://health.harvard.edu

He, X. Z., & Baker, D. W. (2004). Differences in leisure-time, household and work-related physical activity by race, ethnicity, and education. *Journal of General Internal Medicine*, *20*, 259–266.

Hillman, C. H., Erickson, K. I., & Kramer, A. F. (2008). Be smart, exercise your heart: Exercise on brain and cognition. *Nature Reviews Neuroscience*, *9*, 58–65.

Hoehn, C. (2014). *Play it away: A workaholics cure for anxiety.* Copyright-2014, Charlie Hoehn. ISBN: 978–0–615-91817-4.

Hoffman, M. A., Lent, R. W., & Raque-Bogdan, T. L. (2013). A social-cognitive perspective on coping with cancer: Theory, research and intervention. *The Counseling Psychologist*, *4*, 240–267.

Ianzito, C. (2017). Endless recess: The latest trend in adult fitness: Playgrounds. In The *Magazine: AARP.* 18.

Jager, R. F. (2017). CARP Action-Nursing homes going beyond Bingo. In *Zoomer Magazine, 3,* April, 2017

Jansen, C., Miaskowski, C., Dodd, M., Dowling, G., & Kramer, J. (2005). Potential mechanisms for chemotherapy-induced impairments in cognitive function. *Oncology Nursing Forum*, *32*, 1151–1162.

Jenkins, J. A. (2016). Video games aren't just kid stuff anymore. *AARP Bulletin/Real Possibilities, September, 2016,* 8.

Kamijo, K., Hayashi, Y., Sakai, T., Yahiro, T., Tanaka, K., & Nishihira, Y. (2009). Acute effects of aerobic exercise on cognitive function in older adults. *The Journals of Gerontology. Series B, Psychological Sciences and Social Sciences*, *64*(3), 356–363. https://doi.org/10.1093/geronb/gbp030. Epub 2009.

Kasven-Gonzalez, N. K. (2017). Mind and body exercises for brain cognition. Memorial Sloan-Kettering Cancer Care Center. (mskcc.org; brainhq.com).

Kasven-Gonzalez, N. K., Souverain, R., & Maile, S. (2010). Improving quality of life through rehabilitation in palliative care: Case report. *Palliative and Supportive Care*, *8*, 359–369.

Knobf, M. T., Thompson, A. S., Fennie, K., & Erdos, D. (2014). The effect of a community-based exercise intervention on symptoms and quality of life. *Cancer Nursing*, *37*, E43–E50.

Kramer, A. F., Erickson, K. I., & Colombe, S. J. (2006). Exercise, cognition and the aging brain. *Journal of Applied Physiology*, *101*, 1237–1242.

Krause, N. (1986). Social support, stress and well-being among older adults. *Journal of Gerontology*, *41*, 512–519.

Lamberton, D. (2016). State of play. In *Health*: *Chatelaine,* July 2016, 72–75.

Leimanis, M. L., & Fitzpatrick, T. R. (2014). Physical activities and distress among participants of a cancer wellness centre: A community-based pilot study. *International Journal of Physical medicine & Rehabilitation*, *2014*, 2–3. https://doi.org/10.4172/2329-9096.1000193

Littman, A. J., Tang, M.-T., & Rossing, M. A. (2010). Longitudinal study of recreation and physical activity in breast cancer survivors. *Journal of Cancer Survivorship*, *4*, 119–127.

Maddox, G. L. (1988). *Aging and well-being. The 1987 Boettner Lecture.* Bryn, Mawr, PA: Boettner Research Institute.

Maddox, G. L. (2001). *The encyclopedia of aging: A comprehensive resource for gerontology and geriatrics* (3rd ed.). New York, NY: Springer Pub.

McCabe, D. (2017). Rebooting brain science. *McGill News, Winter, 2017/17.*

Oken, B. S., Zajdel, D., Kishiyama, S., Flegal, K., Dehen, C., Haas, M., … Leyva, J. (2006). Randomized, controlled, six-month trial of yoga in healthy seniors: Effects on cognition and quality of life. *Alternative Therapies in Health and Medicine*, *21*(1), 40–47.

Park, A. (2016). Frontiers of medicine: The forgotten side of cancer. *Time Magazine: The View Health,* 20.

Pascal, J. P. (2015). Management of cancer-related cognitive dysfunction—Conceptualization challenges and implications for clinical research and practice. *U.S Oncology*, *6*, 9–12.

Pellis, S. M., Pellis, V. C., & Himmler, B. T. (2014). How play makes for a more adaptable brain. *American Journal of Play*, *7*, 73–98.

Raffa, R., Duong, P., Finney, J., Garber, D., Lam, L., … Weng Jen, H. J. (2006). Is 'chemo-fog'/'chemo-brain' caused by cancer chemotherapy? *Journal of Clinical Pharmacy and Therapeutics*, *31*, 129–138.

Rogers, C., Larkey, L. K., & Keller, C. (2009). A review of clinical trials of ti chi and qigong on older adults. *Western Journal of Nursing Research, 31*, 245–279.
Schagen, S. B., Klein, M., Reijnrveld, J. C., Brain, E., Deprez, S., Joly, F., … Wefelj, J. S. (2014). Monitoring and optimizing cognitive function in cancer patients: Present knowledge and future directions. *EJC Supplements, 12*, 29–40.
Schulte, B. (2014). *Overwhelmed: How to work, love and play when no one has the time*. New York, NY: Sarah Crichton Books.
Weuve, J., Kang, J. H., Manson, J. E., Breteler, M. M. B., Ware, J. H., & Grodstein, F. (2004). Physical activity, including walking, and cognitive function in older women. *The Journal of the American Medical Association, 292*(12), 1454–1461.
Wheaton, B. (1985). Models for the stress-buffering functions of coping resources. *Journal of Health and Social Behavior, 26*, 352–364.
Zarit, S. H. (1980). *Aging and mental disorders*. New York, NY: The Free Press.
Zoomer: Vitality (2017). Brain waves: How to reignite your mind through food, exercise and an app. In *Zoomer: Vitality,* October 2017.

Chapter 3
The Influence of Acculturation and Health-Related Quality of Life Among Chinese Elderly Cancer Survivors

Yasi Xiao and Tanya R. Fitzpatrick

Introduction

Cancer can have a definite impact on a person's quality of life. The diagnosis can cause anxiety and symptoms of cancer can limit activities of daily living. Previous studies have attempted to explain the impact of cancer on quality of life in both the general population and specific subgroups of cancer survivors (Ashing-Giwa, Lim, & Gonzalez, 2010; Ashing-Giwa et al., 2004; Garvey et al., 2016). However, few have studied the relationship between acculturation and quality of life among Chinese elderly cancer survivors. The purpose of this study was to explore the influence of acculturation on health-related quality of life (HRQOL) among older Chinese cancer survivors living in a large city in Canada. The cancer experience of Chinese elderly was explored via each participant's demographic background, language ability, experience with the healthcare system, and general well-being. This study was important because the participants' responses provide further understanding of the experience of cancer among Chinese elderly (Creswell, 2007; Moustakas, 1994). In addition, the results have implications for a marginalized group of Chinese elders by allowing them to recount their story in their own words. At the same time, this research could provide oncology clinicians and social workers with a better understanding of the unique challenges Chinese elderly cancer survivors face in order to access more appropriate services.

Y. Xiao (✉)
McGill University, Montreal, QC, Canada
e-mail: yasi.xiao@mail.mcgill.ca

T. R. Fitzpatrick
Department of Social Work, Arizona State University, Westmount, QC, Canada
e-mail: Tanya.fitzpatrick@asu.edu

T. R. Fitzpatrick (ed.), *Quality of Life Among Cancer Survivors*,
https://doi.org/10.1007/978-3-319-75223-5_3

Literature Review

Health-Related Quality of Life Among Cancer Survivors

Health-related quality of life (HRQOL) is a multidimensional concept describing one's physical, mental, and social well-being in relation to one's health status and disease (Patrick & Erickson, 1993). HRQOL is affected by four components: (1) physical symptoms, (2) functional impairments, (3) emotional symptoms, and (4) social interactions. (Cella & Tulsky, 1993). Cancer survivors usually have lower HRQOL compared to those without cancer, given that they are of the same age and have the same number of comorbidities (Elliott et al., 2011; Weaver et al., 2012). Specifically, cancer survivors are more likely to have limitations on their everyday activities from physical symptoms such as fatigue, pain, sleep disturbances, cognitive impairment, and sexual dysfunction (Naughton & Weaver, 2014). Survivors are also more likely to suffer emotional symptoms such as depression, anxiety, low life satisfaction, and discontent with social role compared to those without cancer. The impact on HRQOL on a cancer survivor is most severe in the months immediately following the diagnosis of cancer. Over time, the mental well-being of cancer survivors tends to improve. However, physical symptoms often persist and, at times, worsen in the years after the diagnosis. Certain side effects, such as cardiotoxicity, from medications also only appear many years after treatment. Therefore, as a result of ongoing physical impairments, cancer survivors' HRQOL can remain low compared to those without cancer (Mitchell, Ferguson, Gill, Paul, & Symonds, 2013; Schroevers, Ranchor, & Sanderman, 2006; Williams, Jackson, Beeken, Steptoe, & Wardle, 2015).

Moreover, some cancer survivors are at risk for a further decreased HRQOL. Existing research suggests there are various different risk factors that could potentially lead to poor HRQOL. Some risk factors identified by multiple studies are young and old age, low education, female gender, poor access to care, low socioeconomic status, low social support, minority status, having one or more other comorbidities, and poor adaptive coping. Often, the survivors with risk factors have lower HRQOL compared to other cancer survivors, and their decreased HRQOL are more likely to persist over time (Byers et al., 2008; Clauser et al., 2008; Naughton & Weaver, 2014; Osann et al., 2014; Weaver et al., 2012).

Cancer Among Immigrant and Ethnic Minorities

The impact of cancer is largely dependent on the cancer survivor's ethnicity and their birth country. Survivors of diverse ethnicities tend to have different experiences such as the doctor-patient relationship, varying degrees of social support, cultural beliefs, education, and socioeconomic class. In general, immigrants and ethnic minority cancer survivors tend to have persistently worse HRQOL and lower survival rates compared to the general population (Du, Meyer, & Franzini, 2007; Luckett et al., 2011). The difference in HRQOL is largely due to increased distress and depression secondary to lack of social support, low socioeconomic status, and low acculturation of the ethnic minority survivors (Ashing-Giwa, Tejero, Kim, Padilla, & Hellemann, 2007; Wen, Fang, & Ma, 2013). The difference in survival outcomes can be attributed to a more advanced stage of cancer at the time of diagnosis in this population. There is an underutilization of cancer screening among ethnic minorities secondary to both lack of access and emotional fears of cancer. As a result, ethnic minorities tend to have a more advanced disease and worse prognosis at the time of diagnosis (Ashing-Giwa, Gonzalez, et al., 2010; Hegarty, Burchett, Gold, & Cohen, 2000; Sung et al., 2000).

Additional challenges are present for ethnic minority cancer survivors that were born in another country and subsequently immigrated to the Western world. Immigrants are more likely to experience communication difficulties during their interaction with healthcare professionals. The poor communication between the immigrant and physician often leads to missed follow-up appointments, noncompliance of medications, and poor understanding of one's illness, all of which ultimately results in poor control of symptoms and suboptimal treatment of their cancer (Ashing-Giwa, Gonzalez, et al., 2010; Butow et al., 2013, 2010). In addition, many immigrants' cultural estrangement with their physicians often results in a poor patient-physician relationship. Cancer survivors feel that they are treated differently and receive subpar explanation and treatment due to their ethnicity (Ashing-Giwa et al., 2007; Butow et al., 2010). Both communication issues and feelings of cultural isolation are sources of emotional distress and culminate in feelings of helplessness and loss of power for immigrant cancer survivors.

Acculturation and Quality of Life

Acculturation is the process focusing on the immigrant's adaption to the host country's mainstream values, beliefs, customs, social norms, and lifestyle (Gim Chung, Kim, & Abreu, 2004). The process of acculturation can be affected by the patient's demographics (age, gender, education, language, native culture, etc.) as well experiences during acculturation such as societal attitude and contacts with the host culture (Berry, 1992). Poorly acculturated cancer survivors often have limited social support and low socioeconomic well-being, all of which can lead to depression, increased mental distress, and decreased quality of life (Kim, Ashing-Giwa, Singer, & Tejero, 2006; Kuo, Chong, & Joseph, 2008; Wang et al., 2013; Wen et al., 2013). This decreased quality of life among poorly acculturated immigrants is largely a result of their limited language proficiency. Language is a critical determinant of health status in the immigrant population. Low English proficiency is often associated with poor health literacy, as language barriers prevent immigrants from accessing information in English (Cordasco, Ponce, Gatchell, Traudt, & Escarce, 2010; Sentell & Braun, 2012). According to the US Department of Health and Human

Services (2016), health literacy is defined as "the degree to which individuals have the capacity to obtain, process, and understand basic health information and services for appropriate health decisions." Cancer survivors who have poor health literacy are more likely to engage in adverse health behavior such as smoking and sedentary lifestyle and are more likely to suffer from mental distress, physical impairment, more intense pain, and an overall poor quality of life (Husson, Mols, Fransen, van de Poll-Franse, & Ezendam, 2014; Sentell & Braun, 2012; Song et al., 2010). Low English proficiency is also associated with poor access to healthcare, as language barrier discourages immigrants from receiving cancer screening or seeking timely medical attention when symptoms arise (Jacobs, Karavolos, Rathouz, Ferris, & Powell, 2005; Shi, Lebrun, & Tsai, 2009; Woloshin, Schwartz, Katz, & Welch, 1997). Additionally, communication difficulties often prevent immigrants from understanding instructions pertaining to medication and treatment, leading to inadequate treatment and sometimes even overdosing (Wilson, Hm Chen, Grumbach, Wang, & Fernandez, 2005). All of the above factors result in more severe physical symptoms and higher mental stress in poorly acculturated immigrants compared to those who are more acculturated (Ashing-Giwa, Gonzalez, et al., 2010; Butow et al., 2013, 2010; Masland, Kang, & Ma, 2011; Yi, Swartz, & Reyes-Gibby, 2011). Although many studies have used language proficiency as the main measure of acculturation, education is also an important facilitator of acculturation. Immigrants with higher level of education attainment are more likely to be well acculturated (Abu-Rayya, 2009; Tran, Fitzpatrick, Berg, & Wright, 1996). Low education itself is a risk factor for decreased HRQOL regardless of one's acculturation status as it is often associated with dangerous health habits such as smoking (Wyatt, Trinh-Shevrin, Islam, & Kwon, 2014). It is unclear if low education attainment can further decrease an immigrant survivor's HRQOL by slowing the process of acculturation. There are very few studies that have explored the relationship between these three elements.

Cancer in Chinese Immigrants and Cultural Beliefs

With a population of over 1.3 million, Chinese is the second largest ethnic minority group in Canada (Statistics Canada, 2016). The existing literature suggests that Chinese cancer survivors are at risk for decreased HRQOL compared to the average cancer survivor. Specifically, Chinese survivors are more likely to have decreased physical, functional, and emotional well-being compared to the general population (Barrett et al., 2016). Cancer pain is often more intense, debilitating and often poorly recognized by healthcare providers. Additionally, Chinese immigrants have higher clinical rates of depression when compared to their Caucasian counterparts (Barrett et al., 2016; Butow et al., 2013; Roy et al., 2005). Like other immigrants, Chinese immigrant cancer survivors' HRQOL are affected by language difficulties and their insufficient understanding of their illness arising from poor acculturation

(Lee, Ma, Fang, Chen, & Youngsuk, 2011; Lee, Pilkington, & Ho, 2014; Leng et al., 2012).

Chinese cultural beliefs, such as attitude toward Western and Chinese medicine, also have a large influence on their HRQOL (Leng et al., 2012). For example, Chinese immigrants are often reluctant to seek medical help due to the stigma associated with sickness and the fear of burdening their friends and family. Additionally, many cancer survivors are dissatisfied with their care due to the general mistrust of Western medicine and conflicting concepts between Western and traditional Chinese medicine (Ma, 2000). Furthermore, within the Chinese norm, the discussion regarding cancer pain and secondary side effects could "distract the physician" and lead to improper treatment of their disease (Torsch & Ma, 2000). Chinese cultural beliefs are more likely to be present and influence the decision-making process of poorly acculturated cancer survivors. Therefore, poor acculturation could further increase the risk of delayed diagnosis and suboptimal treatment of pain that are already present in immigrant cancer survivors.

Acculturation in Chinese Elderly Immigrants

Chinese elderly generally are less acculturated compared to their younger counterparts as they tend to have lower proficiency of English (Mui, Kang, Kang, & Domanski, 2007). Research has also shown that the speed of acculturation is much slower for immigrants that arrive at an older age. Furthermore, in contrast to the typical trend of becoming more acculturated as the length of residency increases, length of time for residency in Canada for older adults was associated with a lower level of identification with Canadian culture (Cheung, Chudek, & Heine, 2010).

Chinese elderly immigrants have similar barriers to health as their younger parts. In general, they are at risk for decreased HRQOL due to their language barriers, transportation difficulties, mistrust of Western medicine, reliance on self-medication, and reluctance to seek medical attention (Aroian, Wu, & Tran, 2005). However, due to the overall lower acculturation level among Chinese elderly immigrants, these barriers are much more severe and prevalent within this population.

There are also additional difficulties that are unique that could further relate to their quality of life. First, Chinese elderly immigrants have especially poor health literacy, as they are affected by both their low English proficiency and their possible declining cognitive abilities secondary to age (Kobayashi, Wardle, Wolf, & von Wagner, 2015; Sentell & Braun, 2012). Secondly, elderly often have transportation difficulties that prevent them from seeking medical help or appearing for appointments (Aroian et al., 2005). For example, they often have difficulties with public transportation and cannot drive themselves. Therefore, the elderly survivors often require their children to interrupt their workday to drive. This further exacerbates the tendency to self-medicate, as the elderly do not wish to become a burden to his or her children.

Summary

Many studies have suggested that Chinese elderly immigrant cancer survivors are at risk for decreased HRQOL compared to the average survivor as a result of poor acculturation. However, to our knowledge, there are few studies that have explored the influence of acculturation on this population's HRQOL. A better understanding of this relationship will shed light on the unique challenges of Chinese elderly cancer survivor and help oncology workers develop services to mitigate these challenges.

Methodology

Design

In order to assess acculturation and quality of life among Chinese elderly with cancer, the *phenomenological approach* in qualitative studies was used to assess the central issues (Creswell, 2007). The goal was to find meaning and further understanding from the participant's lived experience of the phenomenon in question relating to their quality of life. All interviews in phenomenological studies begin with an opening statement. The data collection consisted of in-depth interviews with the participants. In this study, participants were asked open-ended questions that revolved around their experience and factors that influenced their experience. If needed, the researcher probed and clarified the questions to further understand the participant's experience. To analyze the data, researchers highlighted the "significant statements" from the responses and organized the "significant statements" into meaningful sentences that provide context to the significant statements. The formulated meanings were then arranged into clusters of themes that are common to all participants' responses. The cluster of common themes was the basis for understanding the exhaustive description of acculturation and its relationship to HRQOL.

Sample

The sample size included four cancer survivors who fit the following criteria:

- Sixty-five years and older
- Born in China (Mainland, Hong Kong, Macau)
- Canadian Immigrant
- Length of residency in Canada between 0 and 25 years
- A diagnosis of cancer

Table 3.1 Demographic characteristics for the total sample of Chinese elderly ($N = 4$)

Variables	*n*	%
Age (years)		
65–70	1	25
70–75	2	50
80–85	1	25
Average age	74.5	
Gender		
Male	2	50
Female	2	50
Length of residency (years)		
Shortest	16	
Longest	25	
Average	20.5	
Marital status		
Single	0	0
Married	4	100
Divorced	0	0
Widowed	0	0
Education level		
High school	2	50
Post-secondary education	2	50
Bachelor degree	0	0
Postgraduate degree	0	0

The sample consisted of two males and two females, aged from 65 to 80 years with a mean age of 74.5. The participants were diagnosed with colon cancer, ovarian cancer, and lung cancer. The length of residency in Canada ranged from 16 years to 25 years. All four participants were married. Education level varied among participants but none had the equivalent of a bachelor degree or higher. Three of the participants did not speak English or French and identified as Chinese. Another participant was fluent in English, spoke minimal French, and was identified as Chinese-Canadian. Three participants had high school education, while one completed a medical-related degree in junior college. Most of the participants had other co-existing comorbidities. One female participant had poorly controlled diabetes with retinopathy and arrhythmias. One male participant had arthritis and recurrent knee pain that also required repeated visits to the hospital. The second male participant suffered from weakness, paresthesia, tremors, slurred speech, and memory impairment.

It is important to note that two of the participants were married to each other. They were interviewed individually but results may be skewed due to overlapping experiences.

(See Table 3.1 for complete description of sample demographics)

Recruitment and Site

All participants were recruited within the city of Montreal, Canada, via posters. Posters were distributed in popular Chinese pharmacies in Chinatown and community centers such as the Greater Montreal Chinese Family Service and the Chinese Christian Mission Canada. Ethics approval was received from McGill Faculty of Medicine Institutional Review Board and Centre Intégré Universitaire de Santé et de Services Sociaux (December, 2015). In the present study, the participants were explained the risk and benefits of this project and gave both verbal and written consent before the beginning of interviews. Each participant was assigned a number and contact information was stored in a password-protected document in order to ensure confidentiality.

Site

All four participants were recruited via the Greater Montreal Chinese Family Service. This center is a community center that provides resources and services to Chinese immigrants of all ages in order to facilitate their integration into Canadian and Quebec society and to improve their overall quality of life. Some of the services include French and English workshops, interpretation service for hospital appointments, and referrals for difficult psycho-social problems. It also serves as an information center for news updates, job postings, and services within the community. While the coordinators of the center are paid positions, many of the services are provided by volunteers. There is a small fee associated with certain services, such as language workshop and interpretation services. However, for immigrants with economic difficulties, this fee is sometimes waived (Greater Montreal Chinese Family Service, 2016).

Data Collection

After obtaining written consent, a 60-min interview was conducted with each participant. Private interviews were conducted at the participant's convenience in the participant's homes or a private room within the McGill library. The structure of the interview followed the structure proposed for phenomenological studies, which consist of (1) opening statements, (2) research questions, and (3) probes as follow-up to the questions (Creswell, 2007; Moustakas, 1994). During the opening statement, the researchers reemphasized the topic of the research and the strictly voluntary nature of this project. Consent for audio recording, if given, was also obtained at this point. During the interview, the participants were asked a series of predetermined open-ended questions.

Measurement

The key research questions were derived from the East Asian Acculturation Measure (EAAM) (Barry, 2001), the abridged version General Ethnicity Questionnaire (GEQ) (Tsai, Ying, & Lee, 2000), and HRQOL 14 (Center for Disease Control and Prevention, 2016) and modified for this study. The participants were asked questions regarding their background demographics, language, relationships, experience with healthcare system, awareness of social support, and general well-being (see Appendix 1 for complete questionnaire). At times, the researcher asked follow-up questions in order to obtain more information and gain better insight into the participant's experience. This was done if the participants answered a simple yes or no to the question or if the responses were vague. Furthermore, the researcher, while of Chinese origin, was careful not to share any personal experience or family members' experiences with cancer in order to avoid any biased responses.

Data Recording

In-person interviews were conducted with all four participants. The responses were recorded based on the research question. If the participants had consented to the audio recording, the audio files were listened to at home, and participant's response was recorded on to a word document. If the participant did not permit the researcher to audio-record the interview, the responses were recorded on paper during the interview in a notebook, and interview was extended by 10 min in order to allow the researcher to accurately record the responses by hand. Handwritten notes were then transferred to a word document once the interview was terminated to better preserve the data, and the handwritten notes were shredded.

Standards of Quality and Verification

According to Moustakas (1994) and Creswell (2007), the cluster of common themes derived from significant statements must be reviewed by participants to obtain "intersubjective validity." For the purpose of this pilot study, the validation from participants themselves was not possible as two of the participants were away from the country during the analysis period of the study. However, for a full-scale study, the findings would be validated with the participants once analysis is completed.

For this study, a peer-review was conducted with several researchers to review the significant statements and verify the validity of the formulated meanings and common themes. By doing so, the researchers also confirmed that there were no alternate conclusions from the significant statements.

Analyses

In order to analyze and understand the experience of the participants, the *Phenomenological Model* is utilized in this study (Creswell, 2007; Moustakas, 1994).

- Each interview was reviewed and all phrases related to participant's experience with cancer were highlighted and transferred onto a single document. Similar statements were grouped together.
- Using these statements, the researcher developed common themes that reflected the participants' experiences.
- These common themes are then compared to the original list of statements to ensure the themes encompassed all aspects of the participants' experience. Statements that did not fit any of the common themes are highlighted and incorporated into the final report as part of the story of the individual participant.
- A textural description of the participants' experience was developed based on the themes and significant statements.
- Lastly, the "essence" (essential structure) of the influence of acculturation on the quality of life of the elderly cancer patient deduced through the detailed textual descriptions.

Results

In summary, using the steps outlined in the methodology section, four common themes were derived from the interviews: (1) cultural seclusion and social support, (2) general impressions of healthcare system, (3) difficulties during cancer, and (4) general well-being.

Cultural Seclusion and Social Support

Social support for the poorly acculturated participants was minimum. They reported that their children are proficient in English, but their children had moved away to another city or another country in the recent years for better employment opportunities. Therefore, they were unable to provide any assistance or interpretation for the elderly, as their jobs did not permit frequent leave of absences. The only familial social support they received was from their spouses. On the other hand, the children of the better acculturated participant resided in Montreal. Therefore, they were able to provide assistance and support by accompanying the survivor to their appointments or taking on chores around the house.

The participants' social relationships also varied depending on their proficiency in English or French. The three participants who did not speak English or French only had Chinese friends. They could not converse nor express their feelings in English or French (The researcher is fluent in Chinese). Additionally, many of these participants' friends also had low proficiency in English and French. One participant elaborated on difficulties that arose as a result of their inability to befriend English-speaking individuals:

> *We only have other elderly friends. When we need help with translation, we cannot help each other because none of us speak English. For example, our neighbor can speak a little more English, so sometimes she helps us make phone calls. However, if we receive an official letter from the hospital or government, she cannot understand enough to translate the letter for us. We really do want to help each other but we just cannot.*

In contrast, the participant who spoke English fluently reported that she had a culturally diverse group of friends. The majority of her friends were also of Chinese origin, but they identified as Canadian. Additionally, the participant was able to express herself comfortably to all her friends regardless of their ethnic origin. She further explained her relationship with her friends as follows:

> *I think everyone is the same regardless if you are Chinese, Canadian, or even others such as Egyptians. You just have to take some time to establish a relationship with them. When you get to know them, you can all be happy together. I do not feel that there is a cultural barrier between us. I'm friendly with all my neighbors and none of them are Chinese. They always drive me to the metro because they know I cannot walk well in the winter.*

In short, the poorly acculturated only interacted with other Chinese elderly who had similar language, and their children lived in different cities. Therefore, they had very minimal social support compared to the better acculturated participants.

Impression of Healthcare System

All participants were overall satisfied with the healthcare system and the care they received despite encountering certain difficulties. The participants were particularly appreciative of the free healthcare provided by the government. They recognized that cancer is a costly illness and its treatment would have placed a substantial burden on their finances. All participants also thought the physicians and nurses were very friendly. They also believed that their physicians were knowledgeable and fully trusted their physician's professional opinions. This trusting relationship was reported by all participants regardless of the participants' language ability. Furthermore, all the participants emphasized their preference of the Canadian healthcare system compared to the Chinese system. They attributed the early detection of their cancers to the Canadian healthcare system, as they all believed that Canadian doctors are generally more current in the latest medical knowledge and technology in Canada is more advanced. One participant also pointed out that physicians in Canada are very honest in their professional conduct as opposed to the occasional unethical conducts displayed by certain physicians in China.

However, despite their positive review of the healthcare system, participants that spoke little or no English felt that they did not understand or had difficulty understanding the system. These participants described an overall confusion when interacting with specialists. They did not know where to find the specialists needed nor did they know if there are certain specialists that are more knowledgeable. One participant admitted that this lack of understanding prevented her from seeking help even though her symptoms have become very debilitating:

> *I really need to see someone about my eyes. I can barely see at this point. My family doctor gave me a referral for an ophthalmologist but I don't even know where to book an appointment or how to book one.*

These participants also felt that the hospitals offered very few resources to alleviate communication issues. At many hospitals, there were no interpretation services and there were rarely on-site workers that spoke their native language. Participants also reported difficulty accessing the interpretative services at the few hospitals that offered the service, since scheduling must be done in English or French. Some participants who only spoke Chinese also reported a lengthy gap between the first suspicion of cancer to the final diagnosis. One participant reported an 8-month gap between a positive cancer-screening test and treatment, while another participant reported a 12-month gap. The frustrations regarding wait time and lack of resources were not shared by the participant who spoke English. Additionally, the participant who spoke English reported no difficulty navigating the healthcare system.

None of the participants regularly attended any cancer support groups. A participant attended one session of a Chinese support group that she found on her own. However, she found it to be unhelpful, as the session was a lecture on cancer information but she desired social interaction with other cancer survivors. The other participants were not aware of any support groups offered in their language of preference. All three participants who have never attended a support group expressed a desire to attend sessions if it were offered in their language.

Challenges During Cancer

The three main challenges cited by the participants were (1) language difficulty, (2) financial difficulties, and (3) unfamiliarity with geography.

Language and Access to Services

Language was the biggest barrier for cancer survivors who spoke little to no English or French. These participants were able to communicate with their Chinese-speaking family doctors. However, they were unable to communicate with specialists, as it was more difficult to find Chinese-speaking specialists. There were some Chinese-speaking specialists at the Montreal Chinese Hospitals, but they were often not accepting new patients as their patient list was already full. Therefore, all participants had to seek medical help from non-Chinese-speaking specialists and rely on interpreters, if they were available. Without an interpreter, the participants could not describe their symptoms, and the physician had to rely on the physical exam and imaging in order to investigate the illness. These participants also could not understand their physician's explanation or instructions without the help of an interpreter. Unfortunately, there were no professional interpretation services at the hospital where the participants received care for cancer and the participants had to find their own interpreters. As mentioned earlier, the participant's children could not assist with interpretation as they lived in another city. There were volunteer interpreters from the Montreal Chinese community center, but these volunteers have limited availability, as they are generally students and non-healthcare professionals. One participant also felt that the community volunteers provided poor translations as they were unfamiliar with medical jargon and unable to accurately convey the participant's symptoms and the doctor's explanation.

The language difficulty was not limited to the interaction with physicians. The participants' low language proficiency also prevented them from understanding instructions from imaging technicians or questions from the nurses. One participant's wife spoke a moderate amount of English, and this allowed the participant to undergo imaging and blood tests without an interpreter. However, the other two participants' spouses did not speak English or French, and these participants also required an interpreter for simple tests such as blood tests or radiography. One participant voiced her frustration with the inability to access routine tests:

> *The Chinese hospital only offer simple blood test and there are certain tests you cannot get there. My daughter wrote down the answers to the questions they ask before a blood test in English on a piece of paper but the nurses simply will not draw my blood without an interpreter. It really breaks my heart that they are so unaccommodating. They do it to every other Chinese elderly patient who does not speak English/French as well. Now, I just ask my family doctor to check off the items that can be tested at the Chinese hospital so I can avoid going to a French Hospital [...] I know that I need to get the other items tested as well but I cannot ask someone to accompany me every time so I would rather just not get tested.*

As cancer patients, the participants had frequent doctor appointments during their treatment and regular follow-up even after the remission of their cancer. Language issues prevented participants from crucial follow-up appointments. One participant has not had a follow-up in 5 years because she was not able to find an interpreter for her appointments. Additionally, the necessity to find an available interpreter for every single occasion was a large source of stress, although this may be unrealistic. A participant further elaborated on this impact of his language issues:

> *After receiving the diagnosis, my immediate worry was not the cancer itself but the trouble of finding a translator to accompany me to all the hospital visits. Now even if my cancer is in remission, I am constantly worried getting sick again or finding out another thing that is wrong with me and I will have to find someone to come with me to the hospital.*

In addition to the difficulty with hospital appointments and tests, the participants who spoke no English or French also had difficulty accessing emergency services and public services. One participant felt symptoms of a heart attack, but she was unable to explain her situation and her location to the emergency services operator. In the end, both an ambulance and a fire truck were dispatched to the participant's house, but there was a delay since the operator needed to determine the location as well as the nature of the call. Two participants reported an inability to utilize services offered by the government. For example, the public transit system in Montreal offers *adaptive transport*, a door-to-door public transit service for people with handicaps or mobility limitations. However, these two participants were not able to schedule pickups because all scheduling had to be done in English or French. In both of the above cases, the participant did not have anyone in their household that spoke English or French. One participant whose spouse spoke moderate amount of English was able to utilize these services even if the participant themselves did not speak English or French.

The participant who spoke English did not experience any language difficulties. Like the other participants, this participant's family doctor was also Chinese-speaking. However, this participant did not need to hire an interpreter for hospital appointments, whether if it were appointments with a specialist or diagnostic testing. She communicated with her healthcare professionals with ease. She was also able to utilize emergency and other supportive services without help from others.

Financial Challenges

All participants reported experiencing financial difficulties. Three participants retired before arriving in Canada, and their only sources of income were government pension and, at times, some financial support from their children. Therefore, they did not have the financial means to hire professional interpreters or seek help from private clinics. One participant was working at the time of diagnosis but was forced to quit her job due to fatigue. As a result, her household's income was reduced by halve. Financial difficulties were the biggest source of stress for her, and she continued to experience the impact of losing her job 3 years after her cancer's remission at the time of the interview.

Geography and Transportation

The participants also experienced difficulties that arose from their unfamiliarity with the Montreal geography. All four participants reported that they did not know how to utilize the public transit system in Montreal. They were forced to choose hospitals that are close to their house as they required assistance arriving at a new clinic or hospital. This unfamiliarity complicated their experience with cancer, as they felt restricted by their choices of hospitals and felt anxious when they had to travel outside of their geographical area. Most of the participants did not have a driver's license and had to walk to the health facilities.

In summary, all participants felt that they encountered many difficulties during and after cancer but had different experiences depending on their language proficiency. The Chinese elderly who were not proficient in English or French thought their communication issues had the biggest impact on their experience. These elderly also experienced financial difficulties and geographical unfamiliarity with Montreal, but these difficulties were minor compared to their language issues. On the other hand, Chinese elderly who were proficient in English or French reported their financial difficulties as the main source of difficulty. Therefore, issues of acculturation related to language proficiency greatly affected their day-to-day living and well-being.

General Well-Being

All participants' general well-being was diminished after becoming ill with cancer. Participants were asked to rate their general well-being on a scale from 0 to 10, 0 being very unwell and 10 being perfectly well. All participants reported an 8 or a 9 before the cancer. When asked about their general well-being at the time of the interview, the participants reported well-being scores that ranged from 2 to 5.5. The post-cancer rating did not correlate with language proficiency. The participants reported various physical and emotional symptoms that impacted their general well-being. The physical symptoms experienced by participants included fatigue, side effect from treatments, decreased mobility, impaired memory, and symptoms from their other comorbidities such as diabetes and stroke. These symptoms were often chronic, and participants continued to suffer from these symptoms even after the cancer is in remission. The emotional symptoms experienced by three participants that spoke only Chinese included stress, poor self-image, anxiety, and fear of future illness. The fourth participant who spoke English was happy, and negative emotions present during cancer, such as low self-esteem, had improved. The participants who only spoke English were stressed due to the ongoing difficulties with language. Even though they did not have an active malignancy, they had to continue attending follow-up appointments and remain retired or unemployed. Furthermore, the difficulties experienced during cancer were traumatizing, and some cancer survivors lived in fear of going through a similar process again.

One participant elaborated on the ongoing stress and fear caused by low language proficiency:

> *I am constantly worried getting sick again or finding out another thing that is wrong with me. I am not worried because I am scared to die. I am scared because that means I will have to find someone to come with me to the hospital and I have to bother everyone I know again.*

Moreover, many of the emotional and physical symptoms were closely related, as the disability caused by the physical symptoms was the source of stress, poor self-image, and depression. One participant elaborated on the limitation placed by his physical symptoms and the impact it has on his mood:

> *I can't do anything by myself now. I am basically useless. I try to go for a walk in the garden by myself and I fall. I can't write. I can't even pick up a box of Kleenex. Sometimes I can't*

swallow my food. I feel weak and I am just in really bad shape. I am NOT happy. I feel like there is no point to life. I can't do anything, not even around the house. I try to go for a walk and I end up falling in the garden. I sat on the ground for an hour waiting for my wife to come out. I am basically useless at this point.

Another participant who suffers from urinary incontinence shares the impact of this sequela:

This urinary problem is very debilitating. I have to plan everything around it. I have to go to the washroom every 2 hours so my appointments fit around my washroom schedule. I am always stressed that I won't be able to get to the washroom in time. It has become the number one priority in my life.

Although these participants may be in remission and remain as cancer survivors, general well-being continued to be poor.

Discussion

The results of the study revealed three major ways in which acculturation impacted the health-related quality of life of Chinese elderly cancer survivors: (1) low social support, (2) difficulty accessing healthcare due to language barrier that was exacerbated by the lack of resources at sites, and (3) poor emotional well-being.

Firstly, the less acculturated Chinese elderly appeared to have lower social support compared to the well acculturated Chinese elderly. This result supports the association between poor acculturation and low social support demonstrated by previous studies (Kim et al., 2006; Lim, Yi, & Zebrack, 2008). Social support can be divided into two components: emotional support and instrumental support (Cohen & Wills, 1985). Emotional support refers to acts that can improve one's self-esteem or mood (e.g., expression of empathy or love). On the other hand, instrumental support refers to more tangible assistance (e.g., financial support or assistance with difficult tasks) (Cohen & Wills, 1985). The results suggest that poor acculturation is associated with low instrumental support, while emotional support does not appear to be affected by acculturation. All four participants had similar levels of emotional support, as they all had family and friends whom they communicated with regularly. However, the poorly acculturated participants had minimal instrumental support, as their support network was unable to assist with the participant's communication difficulties. On the other hand, the support network of the well acculturated participant provided assistance with mobility issues by offering her rides. The adverse effects of low social support have been well documented in existing literature. Inadequate social support could decrease both physical and emotional well-being of cancer survivors and thus result in decreased HRQOL (Applebaum et al., 2013; Fong, Scarapicchia, McDonough, Wrosch, & Sabiston, 2016; Reblin & Uchino, 2008). The psychological effects of poor instrumental social support could be clearly seen in this study. The poorly acculturated participants felt hopeless and stressed due to the inability of the support network to provide instrumental help.

Therefore, low acculturation could decrease a Chinese elderly survivor's HRQOL through low social support.

The difference in instrumental support is largely a result of the homogeneity of the less acculturated cancer survivor's support network. Poorly acculturated Chinese elderly often befriended other Chinese elderly with similar levels of acculturation, as they share a common language and similar culture. However, it is more difficult for poorly acculturated elderly to develop an emotional connection with those who are more acculturated despite sharing the same language. This is likely a result of their cultural differences, as those who are more acculturated have adopted the host country's culture. Modulating factors of acculturation, such as level of education, may also prevent elderly with different degree of acculturation from forming a close connection.

Secondly, the results suggest that poor acculturation is associated with difficulties in accessing healthcare. Low language proficiency was the biggest barrier to access of care for the poorly acculturated elderly, followed by poor understanding of the healthcare system. Other factors such as finances and unfamiliarity with geography were common barriers to all Chinese elderly in the study. Contrary to existing literature, poor patient-doctor relationship was not a barrier in accessing health in this study. Many studies have found that immigrants, including Chinese immigrants, tend to have a poor relationship with their physicians due to poor communication and a lack of trust (Ashing-Giwa, Gonzalez, et al., 2010; Butow et al., 2013, 2010; Lee et al., 2014; Ma, 2000). Contrary to the above studies, this study found that despite having difficulties in communication, poorly acculturated Chinese elderly shared good relationships with their oncologists. They felt that they were able to trust their oncologists and were very satisfied with the level of care they received. However, similar to the results of previous research, they did not understand the explanation given by their physicians for the most part, which leads to noncompliance and missed follow-up appointments.

The poorly acculturated elderly experienced significant communication difficulties with healthcare workers as a result of their low English proficiency. The result of this study was consistent with the existing research, which has shown that that poor communication is associated with worse health outcomes secondary to delayed diagnosis and suboptimal treatment (Jacobs et al., 2005; Shi et al., 2009; Woloshin et al., 1997). The poorly acculturated participants reported delays in the diagnosis of cancer as they were unable to book medical appointments on their own and the appointment time largely depended on the availability of an interpreter. Participants were also unable to attend essential follow-up appointments posttreatment due to a lack of available interpreters. These barriers could result in delayed recognition or recurrence of malignancy. Additionally, the management of the illness was more difficult for the poorly acculturated, as their low English proficiency prevented them from receiving routine blood tests. This could be particularly problematic for elderly whose treatment response is monitored through cancer markers in the blood (Duffy, 2013).

The difficulty arising from language was exacerbated by a lack of resources within hospitals. None of the hospitals had easily accessible interpretation services, and consequently, the poorly acculturated Chinese elderly either had no interpreters or had to rely on untrained interpreters. Existing research shows that those who had access to trained interpreters had better clinical outcomes compared to those who had no interpreter or used an untrained interpreter (e.g., family members, friends, or volunteers) (Flores, 2005; Karliner, Jacobs, Chen, & Mutha, 2007). In the presence of a trained interpreter, there are generally better communication and better compliance with follow-up and medications. The lack of an interpreter or the use of untrained interpreters is associated with higher medical costs, as these patients are more likely to have more medical tests, more frequent intravenous hydration, and higher risk of hospitalization. Patient satisfaction was also found to be significantly lower with untrained interpreters (Flores, 2005; Karliner et al., 2007). The literature is reflective of the participants' experience, as they also reported poor communication with healthcare workers, dissatisfaction with volunteer interpreters, and poor compliance to follow-up appointments.

The Chinese Hospital in the community does offer medical services in Cantonese and Mandarin, which could alleviate the language barrier for the poorly acculturated. However, the Chinese Hospital is also marred by lack of resources. Participants reported that it is nearly impossible to receive care from the few specialists at the hospitals, as the number of patients requesting for appointments far exceeds the capacity of the specialists.

There was also a lack of resources within the larger community. Specifically, there are no culturally tailored support groups offered in Chinese. There are a wide variety of support groups offered in English and French. However, none of these groups were accessible to the participants due to their language barrier. Many of the participants felt that a support group offered in Chinese would alleviate some emotional distress through exchange of experiences. However, at this point, it is difficult to participate in a Chinese support group due to the lack of Chinese-speaking professionals in the area to offer such as group. Research has shown that support groups can reduce depressive symptoms in cancer survivors and improved quality of life for cancer survivors (Pfeiffer, Heisler, Piette, Rogers, & Valenstein, 2011; Tehrani, Farajzadegan, Rajabi, & Zamani, 2011; Zabalegui, Sanchez, Sanchez, & Juando, 2005). It is especially important to have culturally appropriate support groups, as there are different attitudes toward cancer and depressive symptoms among different cultures. Additionally, various ethnicities may have different prognostic factors and different side effects from treatment, thereby having entirely distinct experiences with cancer (Aziz & Rowland, 2002). The lack of support groups tailored to the needs of the poorly acculturated Chinese could have a significant effect on their quality of life and should be further researched and addressed in cancer support programs and in hospitalized settings.

Lastly, the poorly acculturated participants reported worse emotional well-being compared to the better acculturated participant, while all participants had similar level of physical well-being. All the participants suffered from sequelae of cancer, such as fatigue and impaired memory. Additionally, they all reported symptoms related to their other comorbidities. However, only the poorly acculturated participants reported negative emotions such as stress, anxiety, and fear for the future.

Previous studies have shown that Chinese immigrant cancer survivors tend to have increased emotional distress compared to the general population due mainly to language difficulties (Barrett et al., 2016). However, there have been few studies to address the factors that could explain this increased emotional distress. From the experience of the participants, it is clear that poor acculturation, specifically low English proficiency, is a major risk factor for increased emotional distress. The poorly acculturated participants experienced significantly more stress and fear for the future that are specifically related to their language proficiency and the need for interpretation services. They must continue to search for interpreters for their future medical appointments. As a result, they fear for the recurrence of cancer or another chronic illness that would require frequent medical appointments. Evidently, the language difficulties experienced during cancer were very traumatizing for the poorly acculturated participants as their main emotional complaint was a fear of the lack of interpreters rather than a fear of the illnesses.

Education level may also play a role in the elderly Chinese cancer survivors' HRQOL. Low education attainment is associated with poor acculturation and is an independent risk factor for decreased HRQOL (Abu-Rayya, 2009; Tran et al., 1996; Wyatt et al., 2014). Additionally, Asian elderly immigrants with some college education are more likely to have access to care compared to those with only high school education (Nguyen, 2012). However, the relationship between education, acculturation, and quality of life remains unclear with the study's result as all four participants had relatively low levels of education (high school and junior college). The single participant who had post-secondary education was poorly acculturated and had more barriers to care and more emotional distress. On the other hand, the participants who had high school education had varied level of acculturation, access to care, and level of emotional distress. Future studies including participants with a wider range of education level is needed to clarify the relationship between these three factors.

Overall, the results from this study suggest that poor acculturation among Chinese elderly cancer survivors is associated with low social support, difficulties in accessing healthcare, and a higher level of life stress. Consequently, this population is more likely to have a decreased HRQOL compared to the general population. Their limited language proficiency is the underlying source of these difficulties and can be alleviated with the presence of professional interpretive services.

Limitations

The study's main limitation was its small sample size, as the researcher was only able to recruit four participants in total. The sample size was likely a result of both Chinese culture and the limited recruitment pool. It is uncommon to discuss illness, particularly cancer, within the Chinese culture as it is considered a private matter that would bring shame to the individual if it were to become public knowledge. There is a belief that cancer is the result of "bad karma" or God's punishment for an individual. Additionally, cancer patients often fear rejection from their family and friends after the revelation of their diagnosis (Wong-Kim, Sun, Merighi, & Chow, 2016). This could possibly explain the lack of participation despite elderly individuals showing great interest in the posters distributed at the community center. The researcher was also unable to recruit from the oncology units at the hospitals as the researcher was not employed at the hospitals at the time of the study. Therefore, the recruitment was limited to community centers. A future investigation should attempt to include a larger sample size depending on available funding and access to a wider population of Chinese elderly within the city and the province.

Due to the small sample size, the experiences of the participants may not accurately represent the experience of all Chinese elderly immigrants as they only represent those elderly who were aware of and utilized the community center. There are Chinese elderly who were not aware of the resources offered by the community center as well as elderly who did not require any assistance from the community center. Both of these groups may have vastly different experiences with cancer compared to the elderly who had received some form of aid from the community center.

Implications for Clinical Practice

This study demonstrated that poorly acculturated Chinese elderly cancer survivors are at risk for decreased HRQOL. At the same time, it also suggests several possible points of intervention to improve their HRQOL. Firstly, the result of the study suggests that community and hospital resources should be directed to alleviate the language barrier, since it is a large underlying cause of this difference in HRQOL. An easily accessible professional interpretive service is the most optimal solution for the survivors' limited language proficiency. However, this solution is costly given the hourly fee of professional interpreters. Therefore, this solution would be most feasible in larger community hospitals where more funding opportunities are available. Another possible solution for the language barrier is better trained volunteer interpreters. This solution may be more financially feasible if proper training for medical interpretation could prevent erroneous translation experienced by the participants in this study. Additionally, the presence of professional or trained volunteer interpreters may prevent the unnecessary medical tests that is often ordered when physician do not understand their patient's symptoms. The reduction of cost from the prevention of unnecessary medical tests may offset the cost of interpreters, but more studies regarding the cost-effectiveness are needed in this area. Secondly, resources should also be directed to providing support groups in Chinese. More research is needed in order to identify the most optimal structure of support groups that would be tailored to the needs of Chinese elderly survivors. Support groups in Chinese may not be feasible in areas that have a low Chinese population. Online cancer support groups have been shown to decrease physical and psychological symptoms in Asian Americans (Chee et al., 2016). Research should be directed to the effectiveness of online self-help groups in this population which could be made available to elderly who live in remote areas or areas without a large Chinese population. Lastly, clinicians and other healthcare workers need to be aware of the risk of decreased HRQOL among these elderly survivors. Signs of non-overt distress should be recognized as well, as these patients are often unable to vocalize their distress due to low English proficiency. Information brochures should also be available regarding cancer support programs and resources in the community to further educate Chinese elderly on cancer diagnoses, treatment, and facilities that offer assistance. Available information in Chinese would also assist the survivors to navigate the healthcare system and promote their health literacy, which in turn could improve their HROQL.

Appendix 1 Questionnaire for Interview Based on Modified EAAM, GEQ, and HRQOL 14

Demographics

1. Age
2. Marital status
3. Year of immigration
4. Type of cancer
5. Gender
6. Education level
7. Identity: Canadian/Chinese/others

Language

1. How would you rate your English/French?
2. What language do you speak at home?
3. Do you feel comfortable speaking in English or French?
4. What language do you prefer to speak?

Relationships

1. How would most of your friends identify themselves culturally (e.g., Chinese, Canadian, Chinese-Canadian, American, etc.)?

   (a) With whom do you feel more comfortable expressing your feelings?

Experience with Health System

1. How was your experience with the healthcare system?
2. Do you feel that you have a good understanding of the healthcare system here in Canada?
3. What were some barriers that you encountered in trying to obtain healthcare?

   (a) Was language a barrier?

4. How would you describe the relationship between you and your doctor?
   (a) Do you trust them?
   (b) How was the communication?
5. Did you experience any difficulties during the course of the illness? After you have recovered? If so, what are they?

Social Support

1. How well do you understand the social support or community services that can help you?
2. Have you ever attended a support group?
   (a) If not, why?
   (b) If yes, did you feel that it was helpful?

General Well-Being (QOL)

1. How do you feel about your general health?
2. What are the symptoms you are experiencing?
3. How have symptoms impacted your daily function?
4. How is your energy level?
5. How would you describe your general mood?
6. How often do you feel stressed, anxious, or depressed?

References

Abu-Rayya, H. (2009). Acculturation and its determinants among adult immigrants in France. *International Journal of Psychology*, *44*(3), 195–203. https://doi.org/10.1080/00207590701700537

Applebaum, A., Stein, E., Lord-Bessen, J., Pessin, H., Rosenfeld, B., & Breitbart, W. (2013). Optimism, social support, and mental health outcomes in patients with advanced cancer. *Psycho-Oncology*, *23*(3), 299–306. https://doi.org/10.1002/pon.3418

Aroian, K., Wu, B., & Tran, T. (2005). Health care and social service use among Chinese immigrant elders. *Research in Nursing & Health*, *28*(2), 95–105. https://doi.org/10.1002/nur.20069

Ashing-Giwa, K., Gonzalez, P., Lim, J., Chung, C., Paz, B., Somlo, G., & Wakabayashi, M. (2010). Diagnostic and therapeutic delays among a multiethnic sample of breast and cervical cancer survivors. *Cancer*, *116*(13), 3195–3204. https://doi.org/10.1002/cncr.25060

Ashing-Giwa, K., Lim, J., & Gonzalez, P. (2010). Exploring the relationship between physical well-being and healthy lifestyle changes among European- and Latina-American breast and cervical cancer survivors. *Psycho-Oncology*, *19*(11), 1161–1170. https://doi.org/10.1002/pon.1687

Ashing-Giwa, K., Padilla, G., Tejero, J., Kraemer, J., Wright, K., Coscarelli, A., et al. (2004). Understanding the breast cancer experience of women: A qualitative study of African American, Asian American, Latina and Caucasian cancer survivors. *Psycho-Oncology*, *13*(6), 408–428. https://doi.org/10.1002/pon.750

Ashing-Giwa, K., Tejero, J., Kim, J., Padilla, G., & Hellemann, G. (2007). Examining predictive models of HRQOL in a population-based, multiethnic sample of women with breast carcinoma. *Quality of Life Research*, *16*(3), 413–428. https://doi.org/10.1007/s11136-006-9138-4

Aziz, N., & Rowland, J. (2002). Cancer survivorship research among ethnic minority and medically underserved groups. *Oncology Nursing Forum*, *29*(5), 789–801. https://doi.org/10.1188/02.onf.789-801

Barrett, M., Chu, A., Chen, J., Lam, K., Portenoy, R., & Dhingra, L. (2016). Quality of life in community-dwelling Chinese American patients with cancer pain. *Journal of Immigrant and Minority Health*. https://doi.org/10.1007/s10903-016-0392-4

Barry, D. (2001). Development of a new scale for measuring acculturation: The East Asian acculturation measure (EAAM). *Journal of Immigrant Health*, *3*(4), 193–197. https://doi.org/10.1023/a:1012227611547

Berry, J. (1992). Acculturation and adaptation in a new society. *International Migration*, *30*(s1), 69–85. https://doi.org/10.1111/j.1468-2435.1992.tb00776.x

Butow, P., Bell, M., Aldridge, L., Sze, M., Eisenbruch, M., Jefford, M., et al. (2013). Unmet needs in immigrant cancer survivors: A cross-sectional population-based study. *Supportive Care in Cancer*, *21*(9), 2509–2520. https://doi.org/10.1007/s00520-013-1819-2

Butow, P., Sze, M., Dugal-Beri, P., Mikhail, M., Eisenbruch, M., Jefford, M., et al. (2010). From inside the bubble: Migrants' perceptions of communication with the cancer team. *Supportive Care in Cancer*, *19*(2), 281–290. https://doi.org/10.1007/s00520-010-0817-x

Byers, T., Wolf, H., Bauer, K., Bolick-Aldrich, S., Chen, V., Finch, J., et al. (2008). The impact of socioeconomic status on survival after cancer in the United States. *Cancer*, *113*(3), 582–591. https://doi.org/10.1002/cncr.23567

Center for Disease Control and Prevention,. (2016). HRQOL-14 – healthy days measure | HRQOL | CDC. Cdc.gov. Retrieved 4 December 2016, from http://www.cdc.gov/hrqol/hrqol14_measure.htm

Cella, D., & Tulsky, D. (1993). Quality of life in cancer: Definition, purpose, and method of measurement. *Cancer Investigation*, *11*(3), 327–336. https://doi.org/10.3109/07357909309024860

Chee, W., Lee, Y., Im, E., Chee, E., Tsai, H., & Nishigaki, M. et al. (2016). A culturally tailored internet cancer support group for Asian American breast cancer survivors: A randomized controlled pilot intervention study. Journal of Telemedicine and Telecare. 1357633X1665836. https://doi.org/10.1177/1357633x16658369

Cheung, B., Chudek, M., & Heine, S. (2010). Evidence for a sensitive period for acculturation: Younger immigrants report acculturating at a faster rate. *Psychological Science*, *22*(2), 147–152. https://doi.org/10.1177/0956797610394661

Clauser, S. B., Arora, N. K., Bellizzi, K. M., Haffer, S. C. (Chris) Topor, M., & Hays, R. D. (2008). Disparities in HRQOL of cancer survivors and non-cancer managed care Enrollees. *Health Care Financing Review*, *29*(4), 23–40.

Cohen, S., & Wills, T. (1985). Stress, social support, and the buffering hypothesis. *Psychological Bulletin*, *98*(2), 310–357. https://doi.org/10.1037/0033-2909.98.2.310

Cordasco, K., Ponce, N., Gatchell, M., Traudt, B., & Escarce, J. (2010). English language proficiency and geographical proximity to a safety net clinic as a predictor of health care access. *Journal of Immigrant and Minority Health*, *13*(2), 260–267. http://dx.doi.org/10.1007/s10903-010-9425-6

Creswell, J. (2007). *Qualitative inquiry & research design* (1st ed.). Thousand Oaks, CA: Sage.

Du, X., Meyer, T., & Franzini, L. (2007). Meta-analysis of racial disparities in survival in association with socioeconomic status among men and women with colon cancer. *Cancer*, *109*(11), 2161–2170. https://doi.org/10.1002/cncr.22664

Duffy, M. (2013). Tumor markers in clinical practice: A review focusing on common solid cancers. *Medical Principles and Practice*, *22*(1), 4–11. https://doi.org/10.1159/000338393

Elliott, J., Fallows, A., Staetsky, L., Smith, P., Foster, C., Maher, E., & Corner, J. (2011). The health and well-being of cancer survivors in the UK: Findings from a population-based survey. *British Journal of Cancer*, *105*, S11–S20. https://doi.org/10.1038/bjc.2011.418

Flores, G. (2005). The impact of medical interpreter services on the quality of health care: A systematic review. *Medical Care Research and Review*, *62*(3), 255–299. https://doi.org/10.1177/1077558705275416

Fong, A., Scarapicchia, T., McDonough, M., Wrosch, C., & Sabiston, C. (2016). Changes in social support predict emotional well-being in breast cancer survivors. Psycho-Oncology. n/a-n/a. https://doi.org/10.1002/pon.4064

Garvey, G., Cunningham, J., He, V., Janda, M., Baade, P., Sabesan, S., et al. (2016). Health-related quality of life among indigenous Australians diagnosed with cancer. *Quality of Life Research, 25*(8), 1999–2008. https://doi.org/10.1007/s11136-016-1233-6

Gim Chung, R., Kim, B., & Abreu, J. (2004). Asian American multidimensional acculturation scale: Development, factor analysis, reliability, and validity. *Cultural Diversity and Ethnic Minority Psychology, 10*(1), 66–80. https://doi.org/10.1037/1099-9809.10.1.66

Greater Montreal Chinese Family Service (2016). Mission. Famillechinoise.qc.ca. Retrieved 4 December 2016, from http://www.famillechinoise.qc.ca/index.php?option=com_content&view=article&id=1127&Itemid=29&lang=zh

Hegarty, V., Burchett, B., Gold, D., & Cohen, H. (2000). Racial differences in use of cancer prevention services among older Americans. *Journal of the American Geriatrics Society, 48*(7), 735–740. https://doi.org/10.1111/j.1532-5415.2000.tb04746.x

Husson, O., Mols, F., Fransen, M., van de Poll-Franse, L., & Ezendam, N. (2014). Low subjective health literacy is associated with adverse health behaviors and worse health-related quality of life among colorectal cancer survivors: results from the profiles registry. *Psycho-Oncology, 24*(4), 478–486. http://dx.doi.org/10.1002/pon.3678

Jacobs, E., Karavolos, K., Rathouz, P., Ferris, T., & Powell, L. (2005). Limited english proficiency and breast and cervical cancer screening in a multiethnic population. *American Journal of Public Health, 95*(8), 1410–1416. http://dx.doi.org/10.2105/ajph.2004.041418

Karliner, L., Jacobs, E., Chen, A., & Mutha, S. (2007). Do professional interpreters improve clinical care for patients with limited English proficiency? A systematic review of the literature. *Health Services Research, 42*(2), 727–754. https://doi.org/10.1111/j.1475-6773.2006.00629.x

Kobayashi, L., Wardle, J., Wolf, M., & von Wagner, C. (2015). Cognitive function and health literacy decline in a cohort of aging English adults. *Journal of General Internal Medicine, 30*(7), 958–964. https://doi.org/10.1007/s11606-015-3206-9

Kim, J., Ashing-Giwa, K., Singer, M., & Tejero, J. (2006). Breast cancer among Asian Americans: Is acculturation related to health-related quality of life? *Oncology Nursing Forum, 33*(6), E90–E99. https://doi.org/10.1188/06.onf.e90-e99

Kuo, B., Chong, V., & Joseph, J. (2008). Depression and its psychosocial correlates among older Asian immigrants in North America: A critical review of two Decades' research. *Journal of Aging and Health, 20*(6), 615–652. https://doi.org/10.1177/0898264308321001

Lee, S., Ma, G., Fang, C., Chen, L., & Youngsuk, O. (2011). Abstract B28: Catering to the needs of young and older Asian American breast cancer survivors: In-depth interviews. *Cancer Epidemiology Biomarkers & Prevention, 20*(10 Supplement), B28–B28. https://doi.org/10.1158/1055-9965.disp-11-b28

Lee, T., Pilkington, F., & Ho, G. (2014). Living with cancer: The experiences of Chinese Canadian cancer survivors. *International Journal of Psychological Studies, 6*(4). https://doi.org/10.5539/ijps.v6n4p106

Leng, J., Lee, T., Sarpel, U., Lau, J., Li, Y., & Cheng, C. et al. (2012). Identifying the informational and psychosocial needs of Chinese immigrant cancer patients: a focus group study. *Supportive Care in Cancer, 20*(12), 3221–3229. http://dx.doi.org/10.1007/s00520-012-1464-1

Lim, J., Yi, J., & Zebrack, B. (2008). Acculturation, social support, and quality of life for Korean immigrant breast and gynecological cancer survivors. *Ethnicity & Health, 13*(3), 243–260. https://doi.org/10.1080/13557850802009488

Luckett, T., Goldstein, D., Butow, P., Gebski, V., Aldridge, L., McGrane, J., et al. (2011). Psychological morbidity and quality of life of ethnic minority patients with cancer: A systematic review and meta-analysis. *The Lancet Oncology, 12*(13), 1240–1248. https://doi.org/10.1016/s1470-2045(11)70212-1

Ma, G. X. (2000). Barriers to the use of health services by Chinese Americans. *Journal of Allied Health, 29*(2), 64–70.

Masland, M., Kang, S., & Ma, Y. (2011). Association between limited English proficiency and understanding prescription labels among five ethnic groups in California. *Ethnicity & Health, 16*(2), 125–144. http://dx.doi.org/10.1080/13557858.2010.543950

Mitchell, A., Ferguson, D., Gill, J., Paul, J., & Symonds, P. (2013). Depression and anxiety in long-term cancer survivors compared with spouses and healthy controls: A systematic review and meta-analysis. *The Lancet Oncology, 14*(8), 721–732. https://doi.org/10.1016/s1470-2045(13)70244-4

Moustakas, C. (1994). *Phenomenological research methods* (1st ed.). Thousand Oaks, CA: Sage.

Mui, A., Kang, S., Kang, D., & Domanski, M. (2007). English language proficiency and health-related quality of life among Chinese and Korean immigrant elders. *Health & Social Work, 32*(2), 119–127. https://doi.org/10.1093/hsw/32.2.119

Naughton, M., & Weaver, K. (2014). Physical and mental health among cancer survivors. *North Carolina Medical Journal, 75*(4), 283–286. https://doi.org/10.18043/ncm.75.4.283

Nguyen, D. (2012). The effects of sociocultural factors on older Asian Americans' access to care. *Journal of Gerontological Social Work, 55*(1), 55–71. https://doi.org/10.1080/01634372.2011.618525

Osann, K., Hsieh, S., Nelson, E., Monk, B., Chase, D., Cella, D., & Wenzel, L. (2014). Factors associated with poor quality of life among cervical cancer survivors: Implications for clinical care and clinical trials. *Gynecologic Oncology, 135*(2), 266–272. https://doi.org/10.1016/j.ygyno.2014.08.036

Patrick, D., & Erickson, P. (1993). *Health status and health policy* (1st ed., p. 22). New York, NY: Oxford University Press.

Pfeiffer, P., Heisler, M., Piette, J., Rogers, M., & Valenstein, M. (2011). Efficacy of peer support interventions for depression: A meta-analysis. *General Hospital Psychiatry, 33*(1), 29–36. https://doi.org/10.1016/j.genhosppsych.2010.10.002

Reblin, M., & Uchino, B. (2008). Social and emotional support and its implication for health. *Current Opinion in Psychiatry, 21*(2), 201–205. https://doi.org/10.1097/yco.0b013e3282f3ad89

Roy, R., Symonds, R., Kumar, D., Ibrahim, K., Mitchell, A., & Fallowfield, L. (2005). The use of denial in an ethnically diverse British cancer population: A cross-sectional study. *British Journal of Cancer, 92*(8), 1393–1397. https://doi.org/10.1038/sj.bjc.6602523

Schroevers, M., Ranchor, A., & Sanderman, R. (2006). Adjustment to cancer in the 8 years following diagnosis: A longitudinal study comparing cancer survivors with healthy individuals. *Social Science & Medicine, 63*(3), 598–610. https://doi.org/10.1016/j.socscimed.2006.02.008

Sentell, T., & Braun, K. (2012). Low health literacy, limited English proficiency, and health status in Asians, Latinos, and other racial/ethnic groups in California. *Journal of Health Communication, 17*(sup3), 82–99. https://doi.org/10.1080/10810730.2012.712621

Shi, L., Lebrun, L., & Tsai, J. (2009). The influence of English proficiency on access to care. *Ethnicity & Health, 14*(6), 625–642. https://doi.org/10.1080/13557850903248639

Song, L., Northouse, L., Braun, T., Zhang, L., Cimprich, B., Ronis, D., & Mood, D. (2010). Assessing longitudinal quality of life in prostate cancer patients and their spouses: a multi-level modeling approach. *Quality of Life Research, 20*(3), 371–381. http://dx.doi.org/10.1007/s11136-010-9753-y

Statistics Canada (2016). 2011 National Household Survey: Data tables | Visible Minority (15), Immigrant Status and Period of Immigration (11), Age Groups (10) and Sex (3) for the Population in Private Households of Canada, Provinces, Territories, Census Metropolitan Areas and Census Agglomerations, 2011 National Household Survey. Www12.statcan.ca. Retrieved 4 December 2016, from http://www12.statcan.ca/nhs-enm/2011/dp-pd/dt-td/Rp-eng.cfm?LANG=E&APATH=3&DETAIL=0&DIM=0&FL=A&FREE=0&GC=0&GID=1118296&GK=0&GRP=1&PID=105392&PRID=0&PTYPE=105277&S=0&SHOWALL=0&SUB=0&Temporal=2013&THEME=95&VID=0&VNAMEE=&VNAMEF=

Sung, H., Kearney, K., Miller, M., Kinney, W., Sawaya, G., & Hiatt, R. (2000). Papanicolaou smear history and diagnosis of invasive cervical carcinoma among members of a large prepaid health plan. *Cancer, 88*(10), 2283–2289. https://doi.org/10.1002/(sici)1097-0142(20000515)88:10<2283::aid-cncr12>3.3.co;2-4

Tehrani, A. M., Farajzadegan, Z., Rajabi, F. M., & Zamani, A. R. (2011). Belonging to a peer support group enhance the quality of life and adherence rate in patients affected by breast cancer: A non-randomized controlled clinical trial*. *Journal of Research in Medical Sciences: The Official Journal of Isfahan University of Medical Sciences, 16*(5), 658–665.

Torsch, V., & Ma, G. (2000). Cross-cultural comparison of health perceptions, concerns, and coping strategies among Asian and Pacific islander American elders. *Qualitative Health Research, 10*(4), 471–489. https://doi.org/10.1177/104973200129118589

Tran, T., Fitzpatrick, T., Berg, W., & Wright, R. (1996). Acculturation, health, stress, and psychological distress among elderly Hispanics. *Journal of Cross-Cultural Gerontology, 11*(2), 149–165. https://doi.org/10.1007/bf00114858

Tsai, J., Ying, Y., & Lee, P. (2000). The Meaning of "Being Chinese" and "Being American". *Journal of Cross-Cultural Psychology, 31*(3), 302–332. http://dx.doi.org/10.1177/0022022100031003002

U.S. Department of Health and Human Services. (2016). Health literacy – fact sheet: Health literacy basics. Health.gov. Retrieved 4 December 2016, from https://health.gov/communication/literacy/quickguide/factsbasic.htm

Wang, J., Adams, I., Tucker-Seeley, R., Gomez, S., Allen, L., Huang, E., et al. (2013). A mixed method exploration of survivorship among Chinese American and non-Hispanic white breast cancer survivors: The role of socioeconomic well-being. *Quality of Life Research, 22*(10), 2709–2720. https://doi.org/10.1007/s11136-013-0374-0

Weaver, K., Forsythe, L., Reeve, B., Alfano, C., Rodriguez, J., Sabatino, S., et al. (2012). Mental and physical health-related quality of life among U.S. Cancer survivors: Population estimates from the 2010 National Health Interview Survey. *Cancer Epidemiology Biomarkers & Prevention, 21*(11), 2108–2117. https://doi.org/10.1158/1055-9965.epi-12-0740

Wen, K., Fang, C., & Ma, G. (2013). Breast cancer experience and survivorship among Asian Americans: A systematic review. *Journal of Cancer Survivorship, 8*(1), 94–107. https://doi.org/10.1007/s11764-013-0320-8

Williams, K., Jackson, S., Beeken, R., Steptoe, A., & Wardle, J. (2015). The impact of a cancer diagnosis on health and well-being: A prospective, population-based study. *Psycho-Oncology, 25*(6), 626–632. https://doi.org/10.1002/pon.3998

Wilson, E., Hm Chen, A., Grumbach, K., Wang, F., & Fernandez, A. (2005). Effects of limited English proficiency and physician language on health care comprehension. *Journal of General Internal Medicine, 20*(9), 800–806. https://doi.org/10.1111/j.1525-1497.2005.0174.x

Woloshin, S., Schwartz, L., Katz, S., & Welch, H. (1997). Is language a barrier to the use of preventive services?. *Journal of General Internal Medicine, 12*(8), 472–477. http://dx.doi.org/10.1046/j.1525-1497.1997.00085.x

Wong-Kim, E., Sun, A., Merighi, J., & Chow, E. (2016). Understanding quality-of-life issues in Chinese women with breast cancer: A qualitative investigation. *Cancer Control: Journal of the Moffitt Cancer Center, 12*(2), 6–12.

Wyatt, L., Trinh-Shevrin, C., Islam, N., & Kwon, S. (2014). Health-related quality of life and health behaviors in a population-based sample of older, foreign-born, Chinese American adults living in New York City. *Health Education & Behavior, 41*(1 Suppl), 98S–107S. https://doi.org/10.1177/1090198114540462

Yi, J., Swartz, M., & Reyes-Gibby, C. (2011). English proficiency, symptoms, and quality of life in Vietnamese- and Chinese-American breast cancer survivors. *Journal of Pain and Symptom Management, 42*(1), 83–92. http://dx.doi.org/10.1016/j.jpainsymman.2010.09.014

Zabalegui, A., Sanchez, S., Sanchez, P., & Juando, C. (2005). Nursing and cancer support groups. *Journal of Advanced Nursing, 51*(4), 369–381. https://doi.org/10.1111/j.1365-2648.2005.03508.x

Chapter 4
Ethical Issues in Cancer Patients

Robert D. Orr

Clinical ethics is the identification, analysis, and resolution of ethical dilemmas that arise in the care of individual patients (Jonsen, Siegler, & Winslade, 2015). Cancer patients and their families often encounter questions of an ethical nature. Many of these dilemmas can be adequately addressed by the healthcare professionals caring for that patient. Sometimes, however, the care team or the family may request help from an ethics consultant or ethics committee.

In the 1960s and 1970s, advances in technology caused individuals to ask, "Just because something can be done, does that mean it should be done?" Rules of conduct had to be developed and applied to new technologies. And new technology was very expensive (e.g., dialysis), so huge and growing questions were raised about the cost of care and its distribution. In addition, this was a period of great social upheaval in North America. Major advances were made regarding individual rights, minority rights, consumer rights, and even patient rights. Prior to that, the physician was generally considered the primary decision-maker, but as a result of these social changes, the trump card for medical decisions gradually seemed to pass from the physician to the patient (Jecker & Jonsen, 2007).

During this period of early development of clinical ethics, theologians often asked questions and gave opinions based on their own faith. Over the ensuing decades, the focus of clinical ethics gradually shifted from people who relied primarily on their faith for moral decisions to people who used primarily secular reasoning in such situations. Philosophers, attorneys and judges, experts in health policy, and others became increasingly influential and did much to solidify the

Portions of this chapter have been adapted and modified from Chaps. 1, 4, 5, and 9 of *Medical Ethics and the Faith Factor: A Handbook for Clergy and Health-Care Professionals* by Robert D. Orr, MD, CM, published by Wm. Eerdmans Publishing Co.

R. D. Orr (✉)
University of Vermont College of Medicine, University of Vermont Medical Center, Burlington, VT, USA

T. R. Fitzpatrick (ed.), *Quality of Life Among Cancer Survivors*,
https://doi.org/10.1007/978-3-319-75223-5_4

emerging discipline. And of course, clinicians were part of the discussions: physicians, nurses, social workers, chaplains, and others.

When conflicts were encountered in specific cases, physicians and patients occasionally turned to the court system for resolution. A body of case law slowly developed, whereby legal precedents became established which could be used as guidance in future similar cases. If an individual case was decided in a local court, that decision only applied to that case. If the case was appealed to a higher court, however, the decision then set a precedent for the jurisdiction of that court. Thus, a state supreme court decision would apply to future conflicts in that state; a US Supreme Court decision would set precedent for the entire country (Menikoff, 2001).

In addition to case law established by court decisions and precedents, some issues were taken up by state legislatures. Many states constructed laws about such issues as advance directives, brain death, organ donation, and surrogate decision-making.

Thus, the legal system, both through case law and statutory law, has played a prominent role in establishing precedent and in setting boundaries for acceptable medical practice. Unfortunately, some clinicians and some families look primarily to the law for answers when they encounter specific dilemmas. But as a decisional standard, we must recognize that the law is the lowest common denominator for our society. There are other standards that are more nuanced and more sensitive to common morality. Most often, these standards can be applied at the bedside by the treating team or with the assistance from ethics consultation.

Principles of Medical Ethics Some professionals who work in medical or clinical ethics focus on foundational principles (Beauchamp 2001). It is well accepted that there are four foundational principles:

1. Non-maleficence – From the Hippocratic writings, we have retained the maxim, "First of all, do no harm." This remains an important principle, though it is well recognized that there are virtually no treatment options that are free from potentially harmful side effects.
2. Beneficence – We should do what is in the patient's best interests.
3. Autonomy – Patients have a right to make their own decisions about medical treatment.
4. Justice – We should treat patients without favoritism or discrimination. Thus, if two similar patients have a similar condition, we should offer the same recommendations and treatments to them rather than giving preference to one or the other based on status or our potentially biased assessment of them.

As important as these principles are, there are many situations where two principles are in conflict, and the method of principalism gives no guidance on how to set priorities. For example, it is occasionally justifiable to override a patient's autonomy for his benefit by treating him involuntarily (Beauchamp 2001).

Decision-Making Authority The practice of medicine often seems like an ongoing series of decisions about what to do. Often those decisions are primarily clinical decisions, but sometimes they raise ethical dilemmas. Should the elderly woman with dementia be taken to the ICU for potentially life-saving treatment or not? Should the man with mental illness be hospitalized and treated over his objection or not? Should the severely premature newborn be subjected to painful procedures that have a very small chance of saving his life or not? Who has the authority to make the decision: the patient, the physician, or a surrogate (sometimes called a proxy) for the patient? Such dilemmas are quite common in a patient with progressive malignancy.

Informed Consent It is now a well-established standard that diagnostic testing may not be done and treatment may not be given without the informed consent of the patient or his or her surrogate. Valid informed consent can occur only when a competent decision-maker (whether patient or surrogate) has been given adequate information about the decision to be made and is allowed to make the decision voluntarily, without coercion. There are, of course, emergency situations where physicians are expected to provide life-saving treatment without prior consent.

This exercise of patient autonomy, i.e., self-determination, is foundational in medicine and in clinical ethics. A physician may certainly try to persuade a reluctant patient, but in doing so he or she must not withhold or distort information given to the patient in order to "convince" him or her.

Capacity and Competence It seems intuitive when we say that the decision-maker must be competent, but in reality, application of this concept leads to many dilemmas in clinical ethics. Competence is fairly easy to define but is not so easy to determine. On paper, a person is competent if he or she knows a decision must be made, understands the (adequate) information provided, and is able to use reasoning to assess that information to make a decision that is consistent with his or her values and goals.

Actually, there are two words commonly used for this concept: competence and capacity (or decision-making capacity). Though often used interchangeably, they are not the same. Competence is a global concept – the person is competent or not – and is most applicable in the legal setting. A judge is most commonly the one who makes a decision about the patient's competence. Decision-making capacity, on the other hand, is a clinical concept, and it acknowledges that capacity is task specific (i.e., that a person may be capable of consenting to hospital admission but not capable of deciding about whether to undergo risky surgery), and it may fluctuate (i.e., a person may be capable of making a treatment decision now but may be incapable tomorrow due to changes in clinical situation, use of drugs to treat symptoms, etc.).

Advance Directives The term advance directive usually refers to a written document prepared and signed by a person while he has capacity, explaining to his physician and family what he would want to have done in situations when he might have lost capacity. There have been two basic types of written advance directives, though in recent years, these two components are often combined into a single document.

A living will is an advance directive that says what kinds of treatment a person would or would not want to have in given circumstances. Most are worded to limit treatment and include several vague terms, e.g., "If I am terminally ill and imminently dying with no reasonable expectation of recovery, I want to avoid burdensome life-prolonging treatment and receive only those measures directed at ensuring my comfort." These are good statements of a person's philosophy but are seldom very helpful in making specific decisions. What did that person mean by "imminently dying" – hours, days, weeks? What is their understanding of a "reasonable expectation of recovery – 20%, 10%, 5%? What would they consider burdensome? In an attempt to be more precise, some people include specific instructions: no resuscitation, no ventilator, no dialysis, etc. (Orr 2009). Written statements for full treatment are usually less ambiguous than are those for limitation of treatment.

The primary problem with living will-type advance directives is that the condition encountered is often not included in the wording, or the person may refuse an option while writing about a theoretical situation which, in fact, he might accept when faced with the reality of that situation. For example, many patients say they wouldn't want to be on a "breathing machine." But when asked if they were to develop a severe pneumonia leading to respiratory failure, and the physician felt that use of a ventilator for 2–5 days would allow antibiotics to clear the pneumonia so that the person could return to the same status they had before the pneumonia, many say "Well, of course I would want the ventilator then!" What they had envisioned when they wrote down that they did not want to be on a ventilator was that they didn't want long-term ventilator support.

The other type of advance directive is the durable power of attorney for healthcare, sometimes called a proxy document. In this type, the person designates a person he or she would trust to make treatment decisions if he (the patient) should lose capacity. The person writing the document is called the principal, and the person they designate to make their decisions is referred to as the principal's agent. In addition to naming the agent, the principal may or may not give other written instructions about treatment wishes. In fact, probably more important than signing the document is the actual conversation between the patient and his or her chosen agent. Does the decision-maker appointed understand the personal and/or religious values that might guide such decisions? Does that agent know whether the patient would want resuscitation, and if so in what circumstances?

A patient with any serious condition, especially a malignancy, should be encouraged to formally designate an agent and then to have a clear discussion with that person about his or her treatment goals and preferences.

Surrogacy When a patient lacks the capacity to make a treatment decision, informed consent is still required, but it must be given by a surrogate or proxy. If the patient has named an agent in a durable power of attorney for healthcare, that person has nearly the same authority as the patient. However, for the 80% of adults who do not have an advance directive, for most adults with developmental disability, and for most children, the clinician must identify who is the appropriate surrogate decision-maker.

By tradition, clinicians have granted this surrogacy to the "next of kin." This most often means a spouse, parents of a child, adult children of elderly patients, etc.

However, the concept of next of kin is most often not explicitly defined. From an ethics perspective, the proxy is ideally the person who knows the patient best, is familiar with his or her values or wishes, and is in the best position to make decisions that would be consistent with what the patient would choose if he or she were able. Sadly, but not surprisingly, research has shown that the performance record of such surrogates is poor, minimally better than chance.

Some states have passed surrogacy laws that set out a hierarchy of individuals, based on relationship, who have the legal authority to make decisions for an individual who has lost capacity and has left no written instructions. This is sometimes helpful, but on occasion the person who appears at the top of this generic legal hierarchy doesn't know the patient's values or even has another agenda. There is quite often a more appropriate surrogate than the one legally designated.

Standards Used for Surrogate Decision-Making Once a surrogate is identified, whether as a designated agent, as a state-authorized surrogate, or as next of kin, he or she is expected to use "substituted judgment" in reaching a decision. Some people misunderstand this concept and think the surrogate is to substitute his or her judgment for that of the patient. Rather, it means the surrogate is to substitute a process to arrive at the decision that the patient would make, based on his written or verbal expressed wishes or an understanding of his values.

Only when there is no way to identify the patient's wishes or values do we drop to the lower "best interests" standard. When we have no personal guidance, we try to make decisions that are in the best interest of this patient, recognizing that this is a very poor substitute. In using this approach, we try to determine the benefits and burdens of the proposal and assess what most people would choose in this circumstance. The name given to this standard, best interests, sounds lofty and noble. However, we must recognize that it is the lowest standard we use.

Limitation of treatment (Including Do-Not-Resuscitate Orders) Between 2/3 and 3/4 of discussions in clinical ethics are about limitation of treatment. In the not too distant past, it was believed by professionals and laypersons alike that if a treatment was available, it should be used. Beginning in the mid-1970s, it became evident that many treatments could postpone death, but some of them were only "partial cures." Often patients were saved from death, but left in a condition from which they could not recover, dependent on some type of technology for continued life (ventilator, dialysis, feeding tube, etc.). In addition, some patients chose not to use burdensome treatments (e.g., chemotherapy) that offered some percentage chance of postponing death but also reduced the patient's quality of life during that life extension, preferring instead to live for a shorter period with a better quality of life.

The Karen Quinlan case was the first publicly aired discussion about limitation of treatment (In the Matter of Quinlan, 1976). The Supreme Court of New Jersey set the precedent that it is sometimes permissible to stop what appears to be life-prolonging treatment (a ventilator in this case) when it is clear the patient would not want it. Subsequent legal cases made similar determinations about cardiopulmonary resuscitation, dialysis, intravenous fluids, feeding tubes, etc. These court cases are often referred to as "right to die" cases. This is misleading. There is no global right to die. There is a right to refuse treatment, a right to be left alone. This is referred to in philosophical circles as a negative right. But that does not mean there is a corresponding positive right to be made dead; i.e., there is no such entitlement to death. If there were such a positive right to die, then it would logically follow that others would have a duty to help a person die. This is clearly not the case.

When a decision has been made by a physician and a patient about limitation of treatment, it is important that other individuals involved in the care of the patient are aware of this. The most commonly encountered situation is when a decision has been made to not use cardiopulmonary resuscitation, documented by use of a do-not-resuscitate order (DNR order), sometimes called a do not attempt resuscitation (DNAR) order. This DNR order may be written in the patient's chart in the hospital or nursing home or inscribed on a bracelet worn by the patient. Other limitation of treatment orders include do not intubate (DNI, indicating a decision to not use ventilatory assistance to help a person breathe) and do not transfer to a higher level of care, e.g., don't move the patient from nursing home to hospital or from the hospital ward to the intensive care unit.

Limitation of treatment decisions is very often made by and for patients with progressive malignancy.

Hospice and Palliative Care As these value-based decisions became identified and formalized, the practice of medicine evolved. The hospice movement focused on whole-person care for patients confronting death, including not only the many physical symptoms[1] but also psychological issues (depression, anxiety), social issues (loneliness, unfinished business), and spiritual concerns (guilt, doubt, need for forgiveness). This hospice movement began in the 1970s in Great Britain under the direction of the founder, Dame Cecily Saunders, and then moved to Canada and eventually the USA. Gradually, the field expanded into the more formal medical specialty of palliative care. Palliative care services are a bit different from the original hospice in that the latter are clearly focused on patients at the end of life (generally less than a 6-month prognosis) who are no longer receiving potentially curative treatment, whereas palliative care includes offering services to patients with incurable chronic conditions who may live for some time and/or to patients who are terminally ill but still receiving curative treatments.

Uncertainty Part of the dilemma, of course, is that we often do not know and cannot tell in advance whether a treatment will work or not. We can get some statistical guidance from evidence-based medicine, but statistics will not tell us what will happen in a particular case. Thus, decisions often must be made under the cloud of uncertainty, both clinical and moral uncertainty. Here we must follow the admonition of theologian Lewis Smedes, "When you can't be certain, be responsible"

[1] Though pain and shortness of breath are the symptoms of greatest concern for patients and families, there are a host of other symptoms that should be addressed in a person with chronic or fatal illness, including nausea, vomiting, constipation, diarrhea, hiccups, cough, dry mouth, urinary difficulties, weakness, fatigue, insomnia, and agitation.

(Smedes, 1991). We must make the best decision we can, given the information we have.

Patients I have chosen to refer to as "hospice alumni" provide a striking example of clinical uncertainty. The entry criteria for hospice services are generally a prognosis of 6 months or less to live. And it is generally possible to renew a person's eligibility if they outlive this estimate. In addition, many physicians drag their feet and are reluctant to refer a patient to hospice until they are in their very last days of life. In spite of this, about 13% of patients referred to hospice in the USA each year are discharged because they didn't die.[2]

Another part of the uncertainty dilemma is what does it mean when we say a treatment "works" or "doesn't work?" This leads us into the discussion of futility.

Futility It has become a truism in medicine that there is no obligation for a physician to provide futile treatment. However, the concept of futility is difficult and imprecise. I use the term in its original sense: it will not work, period; i.e., it will not have a physiological effect. Some interpret "will not work" to mean will not have a beneficial effect, and they may mean the ventilator or dialysis machine might postpone death, but since the patient is severely cognitively impaired, it will not benefit him or her. In using futility in this way, the person has introduced a value judgment, almost always using his or her own values. Still others interpret the phrase in a quantitative way. Some may mean a treatment is futile if there is a 99% chance it will not work. Others might set the definition at 95% or 90% or even lower. Thus, even this quantitative interpretation of futility implies use of personal values. The term futility is difficult and somewhat nebulous because it is used differently by different individuals, and it often includes a judgment of value.

My primary concern in the use of the word futility is that it sometimes becomes the physician's trump card. He or she can say, "That treatment is futile, therefore I don't have to provide it." This ends the discussion. Don't get me wrong. I believe there are treatments that are futile, and I believe a physician must have the prerogative to say, "I will not provide futile treatment." However, I think we need to guard against the situation where the physician (or nurse, or other clinician) says "it's futile" when in fact he or she means "I don't think it's a good idea."

Withholding Versus Withdrawing Treatment A generation ago, physicians were taught that it was better to withhold a treatment than to withdraw it. The thinking was that if a patient was being maintained on a treatment, it must be continued. If the physician decided to withdraw the treatment and the patient died as a result, the physician bore some responsibility for the death. Thus, physicians were often reluctant to begin a treatment if there was very little likelihood that it would work. But as more technologies were developed that had the potential to postpone death but leave the patient "half-cured," this concept has been refined.

---

[2]A humorous personal experience is documented in Art Buchwald's 2006 book *Too Soon to Say Goodbye*. New York: Random House.

Further discussion among theologians, philosophers, and clinicians helped solidify the concept that there is no difference in these two actions. In fact, it is now understood that it is ethically better to try a treatment that has a very high chance of not working and then to withdraw it when it is completely clear that it will not work. Withholding it in the first place would have missed those few patients in whom it might have worked.

Conflict Given the complexity of decisions to be made and the vagaries of capacity and surrogacy, it is inevitable that there will be differences of opinion. There may be differences of opinion between the patient and physician, between patient and family, between two or more family members, between physician and nurse, between primary physician and specialist, and the list goes on. Most often these differences of opinion can be worked out through direct discussion, sometimes by soliciting another opinion from another specialist, sometimes by mediation. Rarely it is necessary to go to court for guidance about who has the final authority to make decisions.

There are a few cases in which the ethical issue is between right and wrong, but far more often the conflict is between right and right, i.e., two (or more) options are available, neither is clearly wrong of and by itself, and the decision-makers have to decide which option is better in this particular case. One of the aims of the ethics consultant is to draw some boundaries, indicating that options A, B, and C are "ethically permissible," but options D and E are outside the boundaries of acceptable medical practice, i.e., they are "wrong."

Sometimes conflict seems particularly acute when professionals recommend withdrawal of life-sustaining treatment. They may have been thinking about it for a few days, seeing the patient either not improving or even deteriorating. But they approach the family at a specific point in time to recommend stopping the ventilator (or other means of life support), and the family is not prepared. Even if they have been updated on the patient's condition, even if they have heard the words, they have often not let themselves consider the option of changing goals from survival to comfort. It may require some time; it may require setting some short-term intermediate goals for them to be convinced that it is time; it may require significant support from the clinicians, social worker, chaplain, or personal clergy.

Conflicts often arise because of different perspectives, different experiences, different relationships, different emotions, or different loyalties. But the conflicts that seem to generate the most intense discussion are those based on different cultural values or religious beliefs.

Ethics Committees and Consultants Differences of opinion sometimes lead the clinicians or the family to request an ethics consultation. Hospitals began to form ethics committees in the late 1970s and the early 1980s. Ethics committees originally had three functions: education, policy review, and case consultation. Many hospitals found the process of consultation by committee too cumbersome as it was too difficult to gather the 15–20 members in a timely fashion. In addition, clinicians often found the process intimidating, resembling a quasi-court proceeding, and were thus reluctant to seek help from such a committee. As a result, a large number of hospitals chose to provide case consultation using a subcommittee format. Using this method, two, three, or four committee members, usually from different disciplines, could go to the patient unit, review the chart and speak with relevant individuals, and render an opinion.

The next step in the development of ethics consultation was that some hospitals, particularly larger hospitals, hired individuals to teach ethics and provide ethics consultations. Some were clinicians with additional training in ethics; others were individuals whose primary training was in philosophy or theology who had developed an interest in the medical arena. Because of the diversity in training and preparation for ethics consultants, there is as yet no credentialing process. However, the American Society for Bioethics and Humanities has developed a 40-page booklet in 1998 to help hospitals as they search for qualified and competent clinical ethicists. It was updated in a second edition in 2011 (American Society for Bioethics and Humanities, 2011).

Often dilemmas that present as ethics consultations come about merely as the result of lack of sufficient communication between pertinent individuals. And thus, the resolution may entail gathering those people together in the same room at the same time to listen to each other. In the remainder of this chapter, we will look at several cases in which I have been involved as an ethics consultant. Many details have been changed to protect the privacy of the patients and families.

Case 1

Is it permissible to forego potentially life-extending chemotherapy and stop ventilator support for this patient at the request of her family?

Virginia is a 68-year-old practicing attorney who has been very healthy and has avoided medical care and ignored medical advice until this illness. She was treated 2 weeks ago by an urgent care physician for a respiratory infection, and she reluctantly agreed to hospital admission 9 days ago when the infection had not responded to oral antibiotics. A chest X-ray showed a large pneumonia. Four days after admission, before her diagnosis was certain, she deteriorated and required transfer to the ICU, intubation, and ventilator support. It has subsequently been determined that she has an incurable *cancer of the lung* which has spread to her liver. It now appears that she has sufficient airway compromise from the tumor that it is unlikely she will be able to be weaned from the ventilator without first starting radiation therapy to shrink the tumor.

The radiation oncologist states there is a 40% chance her tumor would respond to therapy (if it is started immediately), and she could survive for several months. Without therapy, he anticipates she will not be weanable and she will likely succumb within 4 weeks. Her family has requested no radiation, and her hospital physician, who has not previously known her, is reluctant to comply with this request since she has a reasonable chance of significant improvement with treatment.

I met with her physician and her close and caring family, three adult children and their spouses plus two of her own siblings. They report that she has always been an active woman who greatly enjoys her family and loves to eat, cook, and travel. Although not religious, she does believe in God; her beliefs about life after death are not known. They also report that she had previously said she did not want to be kept alive with machines, and she has commented negatively about several people she knew who had lingering illness. The family at first requested that radiation therapy not be done. With further discussion, they agreed that starting radiation with the goal of extubation and discharge home was reasonable and in her best interests. They further agreed that an effort should be made to involve her in the decision.

I next met with the patient, family, and care team after the patient's sedation had been stopped. She was alert and appeared to understand the explanation of her condition and the treatment options. She indicated that she did not want radiation, but she did want to go home.

Discussion of Ethical Issues Patients with decision-making capacity should be given the opportunity to make their own treatment choices after being adequately informed of the options and likely outcomes. In patients who have lost decision-making capacity, families can usually give the best estimation of her values and probable treatment choices. They should base their choices on their understanding of her wishes, not on their own preferences. If they decline therapy which the team feels is in the patient's best interests and/or which they believe most patients would choose, every effort should be made to restore the patient's decision-making capacity since some people may make sweeping statements against therapy when they are well but may feel differently when they are confronted with a life-threatening situation.

This patient has clearly said in the past that she would decline aggressive interventions to prolong her life. She now appears to be making a choice that is consistent with that past expression. However, she also says she wants to go home, and this is not an option in her current condition.

Recommendations of Ethics Consultant

(a) Now that her mental status has improved so that she can participate in decisions, repeat conversations should be held over the next day or two with her care team and her family to ensure her understanding of the consequences of her choice. It would be ethically permissible to try to persuade her to accept therapy with the short-term goal of extubation and discharge home, but manipulation (e.g., overstating the benefits or understating the risks) is not permissible.

(b) If she remains steadfast in her refusal of therapy, all other therapies are also optional. She (or her family, if she loses decision-making capacity) could choose to forego antibiotics or other acute interventions or could even choose to stop her ventilator. Since a choice to stop the ventilator would result in significant shortening of her life, that step should probably not be taken immediately upon request. Rather, it should be considered and reflected upon to ensure that it is a clearly understood and confirmed decision.

Follow-Up

After further discussion with the radiation oncologist, the patient firmly decided against therapy, realizing this would preclude her going home, and she further indicated she wanted the ventilator stopped immediately. Her family supported her choices. Her physician felt the patient needed at least 24 h to contemplate this irreversible decision. All agreed on a 24-hour wait and repeat discussion.

I was asked to facilitate the repeat discussion the following day. The patient was sitting up in bed, wearing fresh makeup, interacting with her family, including writing light-hearted messages on a clipboard. Everyone seemed to have a clear understanding of the situation, the options, and the consequences. The patient reaffirmed her choice against chemotherapy and for immediate extubation. I asked her if there were any conversations she needed to have with others, and she said no. I asked if she was ready to meet God, and she said yes. I reviewed with her that it was not expected she would survive after extubation but that this outcome was never guaranteed. She wanted to know about the time sequence, the comfort measures that would be used, etc. Her physician went over the steps that would be taken, up to extubation.

Two hours later, the physician gave the patient injections of morphine and sedation and extubated her. She was given one more small dose of sedation about 30 min later, and she died 35 min after that. An autopsy showed the tumor was even more extensive than had been realized, causing speculation that it would probably not have responded to radiation sufficiently to allow her to return home.

Comment Physicians are often reluctant to agree with family decisions that will shorten a patient's life. Restoring the patient's ability to participate in such decisions will often alleviate this concern.

Case 2

Is it ethically permissible to write futility-based limitation of treatment orders for this dying homeless and friendless patient who wants "everything" done?

Hank is a 41-year-old homeless man who has had a lymphoma and dialysis-dependent kidney disease for about 2 years. He has been under the intermittent care of local healthcare professionals since he was released from prison about 4 years ago. He has been a difficult patient in that he has frequently skipped dialysis appointments, stopped chemotherapy for weeks at a time, etc. His caregivers have been resigned to his "call the shots" attitude but have continued to offer appropriate treatment and provide it when he is willing to accept it. His caregivers report that his body configuration has changed from essentially normal to extreme wasting in the past 2 months from uncontrolled metabolic derangement.

He was admitted 1 month ago with abdominal pain and liver dysfunction, but extensive work-up failed to find a specific diagnosis. He left AMA (against medical advice) 2 weeks later without waiting for prescriptions for his symptoms. The next day he was brought back to the emergency department by two individuals (identity unknown) because of persistent vomiting, diarrhea, and weakness. Since readmission, he has most often refused to talk and has frequently declined nursing assistance. His one point of consistency is that he has always said he "wants everything done," and as recently as yesterday, he repeated this to Dr. Ainsworth, his attending physician, while quite mentally clear. However, Dr. Ainsworth believes the patient is now irreversibly and imminently dying of malnutrition and metabolic imbalance, such that rescue measures (e.g., CPR, intubation) will not work.

The patient has no advance directive, no friends or visitors, and no known family. He has declined a nurse's suggestion that he speak with a hospital chaplain. He identifies his parole officer as his next of kin, but this person cannot be located.

Discussion of Ethical Issues Treatment decisions are ideally made jointly by patient and physician. When there is a disagreement about the use or nonuse of a specific modality, generally the patient's wish for a treatment should be honored, as long as there is even a small chance that the requested modality will be effective. However, there is a long-standing medical truism that says "there is no moral obligation to provide futile treatment." This has been incorporated into professional practice guidelines and hospital policy. The ongoing difficulty is in deciding which modalities become futile at what point in time in a specific case. Sometimes a second (or third) opinion will help to confirm such an assessment or even de-escalate conflict which is not uncommonly generated on this issue. When there is any doubt, the benefit of that doubt should be given to the patient.

In this case, the patient is dying of an irreversible metabolic derangement. Aggressive cardiopulmonary measures will not reverse this inexorable process.

Recommendations of Ethics Consultant

1. It is ethically permissible to write limitation of treatment orders to withhold measures which are truly futile for this patient. Prior to doing so, however, the assessment of futility should be confirmed in writing by at least one other physician besides Dr. Ainsworth.

2. Since the patient has consistently requested "everything," any temporizing measures which can reasonably be expected to postpone his death should be continued.
3. If, however, continued efforts to forestall death (such as limiting his dose of analgesics because they cause a drop in blood pressure) will cause him additional suffering, it is ethically permissible to set aside his goal of death postponement for the sake of relief of suffering unless he has specifically stated his preference to endure suffering for temporary postponement of death.

Follow-Up

Consultation confirmed Dr. Ainsworth's assessment of futility. Dialysis was stopped, limitation of treatment orders were written, and a palliative care consultant advised on end-of-life measures. The patient died peacefully 48 h later.

Comment Healthcare professionals and patients generally work together in developing treatment goals and making decisions about which specific treatments to use or not use. In some cases, however, the patient establishes unachievable goals. In many cases, the professionals are willing to pursue those goals as far as is medically possible, but there comes a point in time when further treatments just plain will no longer work. Determining when the point of futility is reached is not easy. Some physicians are tempted to use "the futility card" more quickly than may be justified because they see the inappropriateness of the patient's choice. However, it is ethically mandatory to set aside that bias and to continue treatment, which may indeed seem pointless, until it is clear to at least two physicians that continued treatment will not have any physiological effect. Then the physician is justified in declining to provide continued treatment, even over the objection of the patient or family.

The patient's social situation, including homelessness, lack of identifiable surrogates, or lack of finances, should not play any role in making decisions based on futility.

Case 3

Should we (may we) tell this Hispanic man his prognosis over the objection of his family?

Alejandro is a 54-year-old man from Guatemala who was admitted 1 week ago for treatment of congestive heart failure and evaluation of thrombocytopenia. He first became ill over 2 years ago at which time he emigrated to the USA to live with family and to receive medical treatment. He was found to have an underlying multiple myeloma, very poor heart muscle function, chronic renal insufficiency, and depression. He is alert and communicative, but he speaks only Spanish.

Dr. White, his medicine resident, reports that his prognosis for survival is 6 months or less, but the patient is not aware he is dying because the family does not want him to be told. Their stated reasons for requesting he not be informed are that it would make him depressed and he would not want to know. This is his first hospitalization. Dr. White believes that the patient has a right to know his diagnosis and prognosis and that he has an obligation to inform him.

Discussion of Ethical Issues In the past 30–40 years, there has been a marked shift in western medicine from the vast majority of physicians not telling patients when they were dying to the vast majority telling patients about their terminal diagnosis and prognosis. Today, there is a consensus in our society that patients have a right to know such information. In addition, most physicians feel more comfortable with the informed patient who participates in his/her treatment decisions. However, the patient's right to know does not automatically translate into a duty to inform.

There is still a very small minority of patients who prefer more paternalistic healthcare and may not want to know their diagnosis and prognosis and/or may want their physician and family to make the treatment decisions without their input. Such patients tend to be older or from other cultures which do not emphasize individual self-determination as American culture does. Thus, patients also have a right to be uninformed.

It is possible that this family is right that the patient does not want to be told of his prognosis. However, it is also possible that the family does not want the patient to know because they expect it would then make their communication with him more difficult. The morally significant item is not what the family thinks the patient wants to know but what he himself wants to know.

Recommendations of Ethics Consultant

1. The ward team should communicate with the patient's primary physician to see if the patient has been informed about his diagnosis and prognosis and/or whether he has indicated that he does not want to know this information.
2. If the ward team thinks that the patient may have incomplete information and does not learn that he has specifically requested to remain uninformed:
   (a) They should tell the family that they want to give the patient the opportunity to ask questions, but they will not force unwanted information on him.
   (b) They should approach the patient (through a medically trained, non-family translator, but preferably with family present) with open-ended questions such as the following: What is your understanding of your illness? Do you have any questions about your treatment? Would you like your family to continue to make treatment decisions, or would you like to participate? Is there anything else you would like to know from us?

3. If it is learned from the primary physician or from the patient that he does not want to be informed about his diagnosis or prognosis, the chart should be clearly marked with this information. While it is difficult to honor such a request in a large teaching hospital setting, it may be workable because of his language limitations.

Follow-Up

It was learned from his primary physician that the patient had been under the care of a Latino oncologist who had told him that he had an infection in his bone marrow that required periodic regular treatment with intravenous medication. He was not aware of his prognosis. Dr. White sat down with the patient, with his family present, and through a hospital translator told him about his current test results and status and asked him: (a) "Has anyone told you what to expect from this disease?" His answer, "No." (b) "Do you want to know what is likely to happen, or would you rather just wait and see what happens?" Answer, "I'd rather wait and see." (c) "Do you want your family and doctors to continue to make treatment decisions, or would you like to be consulted?" Answer, "You can talk with them."

Comment When faced with situations like this, we may be tempted to feel culturally superior, believing that we have advanced to a higher plane. However, the role of family in protecting patients from bad things, including bad news, is an important cultural value that we shouldn't ignore. It is probably true in those situations, as it was in our own culture prior to the changes in the 1960s, that patients really do know or suspect their poor prognosis, but if they do not expect to be informed, it is culturally arrogant for us to force this information on them. There may be an occasional situation where major decisions must be made with significant trade-offs of survival, disability, etc. in which we should strongly encourage patient participation. But if the patient indicates a desire for others to make such decisions, we should honor that choice.

Case 4

Is it ethically permissible for this 11-year-old child's parents to forego potentially life-saving treatment for her malignancy?

Jennifer, age 11, was found 6 months ago to have an osteosarcoma in her femur which was felt to have a 75% chance of cure with vigorous therapy. She was evaluated at a large children's hospital. Upon specialist recommendation, she received and tolerated 6 weeks of preliminary chemotherapy given by Dr. Martin, a pediatric oncologist in this community. Though her parents initially preferred amputation, they were persuaded to return to the children's hospital for limb-salvage surgery

2 months ago. This surgery has a much better functional result than amputation. Unfortunately, the pathology report showed the tumor to be more advanced than originally suspected, suggesting that her prognosis for survival would be reduced to 40–50%. Standard therapy is that she should now receive 6 months of follow-up chemotherapy.

Her parents are considering foregoing further chemotherapy based on their belief that she is dying and the chemotherapy is too toxic. The proposed drug has a low incidence of brain toxicity; however this side effect is only seen when the drug is used in higher doses than she would receive.

Her parents openly talk about her death in front of her. All her professional caregivers here and at the children's hospital believe it is clearly in the child's best interests to have the chemotherapy since her prognosis for long-term survival without it is near zero. Though her parents have not made a definitive refusal of further therapy, they have been postponing meetings, discussions, and a decision, and her prognosis worsens with such delays.

Jennifer was adopted as an infant, but her well-educated and well-read parents are convinced that she has not assimilated well into their family. She has been in counseling and on sedating medication for 2 or 3 years. Her parents are concerned that she has a baseline defect in cognitive function, and they fear the chemotherapy may cause further brain damage.

Discussion of Ethical Issues Parents have the right to make treatment decisions for their child and the responsibility to act in her best interests. Since a child's "best interests" are not easily defined, and since not all parents will come to identical decisions in similar situations, our society allows parents some ill-defined degree of discretion in making treatment decisions.

Physicians have the responsibility to recommend to parents what they believe to be in a child's best interests. That recommendation should be based on the best available data and, in cases of doubt, should include consultation and/or second opinion. Physicians likewise have the responsibility to oversee the scope of parental discretion. They are expected to notify Child Protective Services if parents are making a choice that is clearly outside a "reasonable construal of the child's best interests."

In this case, there is strong professional agreement on what treatment is in this child's best interests. Her parents are postponing a semi-urgent treatment decision, and they have demonstrated attitudes and behavior suggesting they may not be seeking her best interests.

Recommendations of Ethics Consultant

Since there is a strong professional consensus that further therapy offers significant life-prolonging benefit for this patient:

1. Dr. Martin should:
   - Document the joint recommendation for further treatment
   - Inform the parents again, in person and/or via registered mail, of this joint recommendation and the urgency of beginning therapy
2. If the parents do not agree to begin therapy within a clearly specified time, Child Protective Services should be notified of your concerns about medical neglect.

Follow-Up

Dr. Martin sent a certified letter to her parents saying chemotherapy should begin within 7 days, and failure to do so would necessitate a report to Child Protective Services. After another frustrating delay, Jennifer was admitted for the chemotherapy. Unfortunately, a chest X-ray done at that time showed that the cancer had spread to her lungs, making cure impossible. The new tumors had probably been present for several weeks, so earlier initiation of chemotherapy would not likely have made an ultimate difference.

Comment Respect for family integrity and protection of vulnerable children are both important societal values. When they appear to conflict, it is often very difficult to know when is the appropriate time to use the agencies of society to intervene. Such was the case here. The oncologist's approach in this case was that of trying to work with the parents to find a reasonable approach that would meet their goals and protect the child's best interests. What eventually became clear was that Jennifer's parents seemed to be preparing themselves (and her) for her death before it was clear that she would not survive. Once this became clear, there was no option except to bring external forces to bear to make them move forward quickly. Unfortunately, even this did not allow her to reach the hoped for outcome.

Conclusions

Patients with malignancies and their families often confront difficult decisions, some purely clinical, others with ethical dimensions. It should be the goal of all healthcare professionals to assist them in making the decision that is consistent with good medical care and also consistent with the patient's values. Rarely are such decisions black or white. Each case is unique. Including an ethics consultant or committee may, in some cases, help determine what is the "best" decision for a particular patient.

References

American Society for Bioethics and Humanities. (2011). *Core competencies for health care ethics consultation*. Chicago, IL: ASBH.

Beauchamp, T. L., & Childress, J. F. (2001). *Principles of medical ethics* (5th ed.). New York, NY: Oxford University Publishers.

In the matter of Karen Quinlan.(1976). 70 N.J. 10, 335 A. 2d 647.

Jecker, N., & Jonsen, A. R. (2007). *Bioethics: Introduction to history, methods, and practice* (2nd ed.). Sudbury, MA: Jones and Bartlett Publishers.

Jonsen, A. R., Siegler, M., & Winslade, W. J. (2015). *Clinical ethics* (8th ed.). New York, NY: McGraw-Hill.

Menikoff, J. (2001). *Law and bioethics: An introduction*. Washington, DC: Georgetown University Press.

Orr, R.D. (2009). *Medical ethical and the faith factor: A handbook for clergy and health-care professionals*. Grand Rapids, MI: Wm. B. Eerdmans Publishing.

Smedes, L. (1991). *Choices: Making right decisions in a complex world*. New York, NY: Harper Collins.

Additional References on the Ethical Foundation of Medicine

American Medical Association's Council on Ethical and Judicial Affairs. (2005). *Code of medical ethics 2004–2005: Current opinions with annotations*. Chicago, IL: American Medical Association.

Campbell, A., Gillett, G., & Jones, G. (2001). *Medical ethics* (3rd ed.). Oxford, UK: Oxford University Press.

Engelhardt, H. T. (1996). *The foundations of bioethics* (2nd ed.). New York, NY: Oxford University Press.

Gert, B. (2006). *Bioethics* (2nd ed.). Oxford, UK: Oxford University Press.

Lo, B. (2013). *Resolving ethical dilemmas: A guide for clinicians* (5th ed.). Philadelphia, PA: Lippincott Williams & Wilkins.

Chapter 5
Genetic Mutations in Cancer Susceptibility Genes: A Family History of Cancer

Janice L. Berliner and Megan Harlan Fleischut

Introduction

Hereditary Breast Cancer

For many years, there were only two known genes having to do with hereditary breast cancer, called BRCA1 and BRCA2. Clinical testing has been available for these genes since 1996, and well over 2 million people have been tested to see if they carry *BRCA* mutations (Myriad Genetic Laboratories, 2017). These mutations significantly increase the risk for breast cancer in both men and women as well as ovarian cancer in women, and somewhat increase the risk for prostate cancer in men and pancreatic cancer in both men and women (Chen & Parmigiani, 2007; Mavaddat et al., 2013; Mersch et al., 2015).

Over the past several years, more genes have been discovered that, when mutated, also increase the risks for breast and/ovarian cancer (Easton, et al., 2007; Rahman et al., 2007; Renwick et al., 2006; Walsh & King, 2007; Walsh et al., 2011). Due to the development of next-generation sequencing techniques, panel testing is now widely available to test many genes simultaneously, avoiding the need for sequential testing of genes and waiting for results each time. All of this is carefully explained by Shelly (the genetic counselor) to her patient Bella, and many issues are raised in the process.

Bella is a 35-year-old woman of Italian descent who arrives at the genetics clinic at the recommendation of her medical oncologist, Dr. S, full of concern and anxiety. Given her recent diagnosis of early-onset breast cancer, the doctor asks her some

J. L. Berliner (✉)
Memorial Sloan Kettering Cancer Center, Clinical Genetics Service, Basking Ridge, NJ, USA
e-mail: berlinej@mskcc.org

M. H. Fleischut
Memorial Sloan Kettering Cancer Center, Clinical Genetics Service, New York, NY, USA
e-mail: harlanm@mskcc.org

T. R. Fitzpatrick (ed.), *Quality of Life Among Cancer Survivors*,
https://doi.org/10.1007/978-3-319-75223-5_5

pointed questions about her family history, and Bella reveals that while her mother and the rest of her maternal family history are unaffected by cancer and everyone passed away from heart disease, her father's side of the family is "riddled with cancer." Bella admits that she always felt it was only a matter of time until it hit her too, although a small part of her held out hope that since it was on her father's side of the family it might not affect her. She provides the details that her paternal aunt had been diagnosed with breast cancer in her 40s and died soon after, a first cousin had been diagnosed with breast cancer at 52 years but happily was doing well after surgery and chemotherapy at age 55, and her paternal grandmother had died from some form of "woman's cancer" in her late 30s but no one in the family could really figure it out. She says her father remembers his mother having had a full hysterectomy when he was a child, so his assumption was that it was an ovarian cancer, but Dr. S points out that a hysterectomy would also likely have been performed for a uterine or cervical cancer as well. At this point, Dr. S feels strongly that there is enough in the family to recommend that Bella see a genetic counselor for risk assessment, an explanation of her options for genetic testing, and a thorough discussion of what genetic test results might mean for Bella and her family members. Bella tearfully tells Dr. S that she is mostly concerned for her sister, as she herself has already been diagnosed. "The cow's out of the barn for me" she says; "please help me find a way to protect my sister so she doesn't have to go through this too."

For the week leading up to Bella's appointment, she speaks with friends and colleagues about her concerns. How will the appointment with the genetic counselor go? What will she be tested for? What would the results tell her? Would her sister develop cancer too? What if she wanted to have another baby – would she be able to? What about her daughter – would her cancer risk be high too? She doesn't sleep so well that week, as her conversations with friends and Google searches give her conflicting information and raise more questions than they answer.

Pretest Genetic Counseling

When the day arrives to meet with the genetic counselor, Bella feels both relieved and nervous. She needs her questions answered but fears she will hear some scary news. She doesn't want to be told that she shouldn't have another child because he or she would be at high risk for cancer or that her sister should have her breasts removed to avoid developing breast cancer like she did. This is all too much. "Maybe I'll just cancel the appointment," she says out loud more than once throughout the week. But the answer she gives herself is that knowledge is power and she will be better off being in control than in the dark. So she takes a deep breath and walks into the genetics clinic at the appointed hour to meet with Shelly, her genetic counselor. What she finds in Shelly is a genuinely empathic, compassionate, good listener who starts by asking her what her primary concerns are and how she can be of help, putting her at ease right away. Bella describes her family history as Shelly takes copious notes and draws a detailed family tree. Shelly verifies with Bella that she

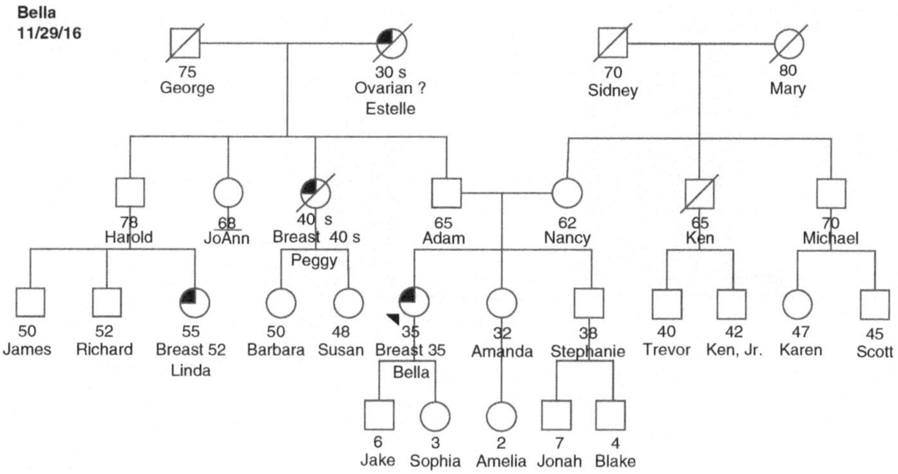

Fig. 5.1 Bella's family tree

has drawn it correctly and then asks her if there is any way to obtain medical records or pathology reports from her grandmother's diagnosis, as it would be helpful to confirm what type of cancer she had. Even a death certificate might have this information, and Bella says she will try to track it down (Fig. 5.1).

Bella tells Shelly what she had said to Dr. S – that she had known that cancer would affect her at some point, given her family history. Shelly explains that, in fact, a large majority of cancers are actually NOT hereditary, despite the media hype (Schrader et al., 2016; Zhang et al., 2015). Having an affected mother with breast cancer does not doom one to that fate, just like having a mother free from breast cancer does not protect one from it. She goes on to explain that we have two copies of every gene, one from each parent. Cancer genes are almost always inherited in a dominant fashion, such that they only need to be inherited from one parent in order for the individual to be predisposed to cancer. However, cancer does not develop until/unless the other copy of the gene (inherited from the other parent) becomes mutated at a later time in life for reasons that are still unknown. This second event is not hereditary but happens because of some environmental or other triggers.

Cancer Risks in Those Already Diagnosed as Well as Unaffected Family Members

Bella arrives at Shelly's office saying that she has two big concerns: the first is the likelihood that her cancer will come back, and the second is about her sister's cancer risks. Shelly points out to Bella that there is an important difference between recurrence of her current cancer and the development of a new cancer. Recurrence is a result of the grade and stage of the cancer, how the disease is treated, and how

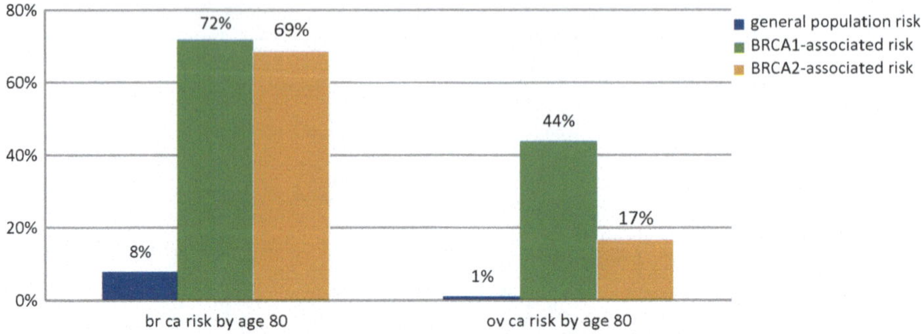

Fig. 5.2 Breast and ovarian cancer risks related to *BRCA* mutations (Source: Kuchenbaecker et al., 2017)

the body reacts to the treatment. It is an oncology issue, not a genetics issue. At the same time, having already been diagnosed with cancer does not protect her against developing another new cancer in the future. This risk is fairly difficult to calculate without knowing whether Bella carries a mutation in a hereditary breast and/or ovarian cancer gene. So Shelly embarks upon a comprehensive discussion of the various genes known to be associated with breast and ovarian cancer and what Bella could do with the test results once she has them vis-à-vis cancer screening and/or preventative surgeries. She carefully explains that there are both high-risk genes, such as BRCA1 and BRCA2, and moderate-risk genes. *BRCA1* and *BRCA2*, when mutated, are known to increase a woman's breast and ovarian cancer risk quite substantially, as shown in Fig. 5.2 (Kuchenbaecker et al., 2017).

There are other high-risk genes that not only raise the risks for breast and/or ovarian cancer but can also raise the risks for other forms of cancer, although these risks are less well-defined (Couch et al., 2017; Tung et al., 2016). There are also some moderate-risk genes that, when mutated, likely contribute to the development of cancer but probably do not, by themselves, cause cancer (see Table 5.1). The environment, other modifying genes, and random chance likely play a role as well.

As Shelly explains all these details, Bella begins to realize how complicated genetic testing for cancer genes really is. She had thought that she would just have blood drawn and in a week or two she would know if her cancer was something she inherited from her dad's side of the family. As they keep talking, many questions start bubbling up in Bella's head, but the first of them is what is the likelihood that her sister or her daughter will have breast cancer too? Shelly quickly reminds Bella that the vast majority of cancers are not hereditary and that if Bella does not have a mutation in a hereditary cancer gene, it would be very reassuring. It would not guarantee that her sister and daughter are not at increased risk because not all cancer genes have been discovered yet, but it would certainly lower the risks substantially.

After a long discussion of the cancer risks associated with various gene mutations, what Bella might be able to do to protect her health if she were found to have a mutation, and which family members may also be at risk if a mutation were to run

Table 5.1 High or moderate risk gene, syndrome and linked cancer

Gene(s)	High- or moderate-risk gene(s)	Syndrome name (if any)	Major linked cancers
BRCA1 *BRCA2*	High	Hereditary breast-ovarian cancer syndrome	Breast Ovarian Pancreas Prostate
TP53	High	Li-Fraumeni syndrome	Breast Sarcoma Leukemia Brain Adrenal Possible other sites
PTEN	High	Cowden syndrome	Breast Uterine Thyroid Colon Kidney
ATM	Moderate	None	Breast Pancreatic*
CHEK2	Moderate	None	Breast Colon*
PALB2	Moderate	None	Breast Pancreatic* Ovarian*
RAD51C *RAD51D*	Moderate	None	Ovarian
BRIP1	Moderate	None	Ovarian
MLH1 *MSH2* *MSH6* *PMS2* *EPCAM*	High	Lynch syndrome	Colon Uterine Ovarian Stomach Small intestine Urinary tract Pancreatic Possible other sites

Source: Memorial Sloan Kettering Cancer Center Clinical Genetic Service
*For these cancers, the link between the gene and cancer is uncertain

in the family, Bella opts to have genetic testing. She signs the informed consent forms and has her blood drawn and talks with Shelly about turnaround time for the results and how the results will be disclosed to her. Shelly explains that she will meet with Bella again once the results are ready so that they can have a thorough conversation about what the results mean, even if she does not have a mutation. There is even a possibility of having a result called a variant of uncertain significance, where a segment of DNA in one of the genes is identified that is not the normal sequence of DNA but is not known to be a mutation either. In these cases, Shelly explains, there is no current understanding of the meaning of the result, and no changes in her medical management would be recommended. No other family members would be offered genetic testing because not understanding it in Bella would mean not understanding it in the family members either, at least not currently.

Results Disclosure

After an emotional three weeks of waiting and wondering, Bella returns to the genetic counseling clinic to meet again with Shelly. She is hoping for the best but preparing for the worst. She has fairly well convinced herself that she will have a mutation, as she would rather be pleasantly surprised if it is negative than devastated if it is positive. She has admitted this to her husband, who holds her hand tightly as they follow Shelly from the waiting room into her office. He gives her hand a squeeze and smiles at her briefly as they sit down across from Shelly. Shelly starts by saying that she understands it has probably been a bit tough to wait for the results and asks if Bella and her husband, Jake, have any questions before she begins. They don't, so she begins by saying that indeed a mutation within the *BRCA2* gene was found. She pauses for several seconds to determine if this information has registered with Bella and Jake and asks if Bella remembers what that means. Bella wipes away a tear and quietly says she remembers that now her ovarian cancer risk goes up and she should have her ovaries removed. Shelly asks if Bella and Jake have thought about having any more children. They look at each other. Jake answers that they had been talking about it, but then Bella was diagnosed with breast cancer, and their plans were put on hold.

Reproductive Options

Bella and Jake were told by the oncologist that if she needs chemotherapy that this will likely make her periods stop, so that if they would like to have more children they could consider having some of her eggs retrieved and stored. Shelly also points out that with *BRCA2* mutations, while the ovarian cancer risk certainly is increased over the background population risk, the risk does not begin to increase sharply until a little later. That means that Shelly could consider putting off the surgery until she is 40 but that it is the standard of care for BRCA carriers to have their ovaries and fallopian tubes removed due to the lack of reliable screening for ovarian cancer. There are available screening measures, but none are thought to reduce the risk of death from ovarian cancer (Buys et al., 2011).

Another option to consider if Bella and Jake would like to have more children is called preimplantation diagnosis or PGD. This is helpful for those who would prefer not to pass the mutation on to the next generation but would rather not have to face the decision of whether to terminate a pregnancy, as is the decision when diagnosed with either amniocentesis or chorionic villus sampling (CVS). Each child of a mutation carrier has a 50% chance to inherit the mutation and of course a 50% chance not to. PGD allows the conception of an unaffected pregnancy in the first place; embryos are created in the laboratory by in vitro fertilization and safely removing a cell from the embryo to test it for the presence of the *BRCA* mutation (Lee, Chow, Yeung, & Ho, 2017; Offit et al., 2006; Sagi et al., 2009). If the embryo is affected, it is not implanted in the uterus, and if it is unaffected, it is. This avoids even the consideration of pregnancy termination because only unaffected embryos are utilized.

Shelly asks Bella and Jake if this is something they would consider and is met with nervous laughter. "Well," Bella starts slowly, "I never knew that was thing! I mean, we weren't sure if we were going to have another child, and our heads have been reeling anyway since Dr. S told us I might lose my fertility due to the chemo. Now you tell us we might be able to have a child and think about having him or her not carry this mutation. That's a lot to swallow all at once." She glances at Jake who is nodding his head in agreement. She looks back at Shelly, who is smiling.

"It IS a lot," Shelly agrees, "but it's also a possibility for you. Just think about it. It's nothing you need to decide right now and you can talk to me anytime if you have questions. And in fact, I'll refer you to one of my genetic counseling colleagues who specializes in assisted reproductive technologies so that you can speak with her for more details. Okay?" Bella and Jake are happy to take her up on that offer, and Shelly asks them for their permission to move on to another important topic for their visit.

Breast Cancer Risk and Options for Surveillance and Surgery

Shelly asks Bella what else, if anything, she remembers from their pre-test session about her cancer risks. Bella says she knows that *BRCA* mutations increase the risks for breast and ovarian cancer but that she's already had breast cancer so she figures she's not too worried about that one. Again, Jake nods in agreement. Shelly sighs to herself, as she hears this from many of her patients and wonders why this part is lost in translation so often. She takes a deep breath and begins. "Bella, I know this is scary. I know that after having been told once that you have breast cancer that the very last thing in the world you ever want to hear is those words again. However, in the interest of your safety I have to remind you that having a *BRCA2* mutation not only explains where your first breast cancer diagnosis came from, but also raises the likelihood that you could develop a new breast cancer in the future. For this reason, you can consider extra surveillance measures, such as a breast MRI each year in addition to your annual mammogram, or you could consider having a bilateral preventative mastectomy." She hears Bella suck in her breath. "You don't need to decide anything right now," Shelly continues. "In fact, I would encourage you to meet with a plastic surgeon to discuss what your reconstructive options would be before making any decisions at all."

"When would I need to do this?" Bella asks. "When would I need to start screening or have surgery?"

"Well, your doctors are going to watch you very carefully, given your current diagnosis. You're going to be having scans during your treatment and if you follow your doctors' recommendations for now, that's perfectly fine." Shelly smiles in support for Bella and Jake. "But since a mammogram will be part of your screening plan each year, you can also have a breast MRI, and most doctors will recommend that they are staggered 6 months apart."

"Okay," Jake interjects "that makes sense for Bella, and I want to make sure that she's protected as much as possible, but what about our kids?"

Concern for Family Members

"I'm glad you asked that question," Shelly says. "Your kids are very young, and while I'd be a fool to tell you not to worry about your children because as parents we all worry, this makes it much easier. It will probably be twenty five to thirty years before they are at increased risk for cancer, and this is only if they inherited Bella's *BRCA2* mutation in the first place. Remember from our earlier discussion that there is a 50% chance for each of them to have the mutation and 50% not to. If they do, then their risks would be increased, but not for many years, by which time our medical landscape will look very different and our methods of detection, treatment and even prevention will be vastly different. The bigger concern, currently, is your sister and brother. They have the same 50% probability of having the mutation that your children do, but their cancer risks if they do have it would be much sooner. So screening and/or surgery, particularly for your sister, would be important considerations. I would certainly encourage them to come in for their own genetic counseling and testing as soon as they feel ready. Your aunts, uncles and cousins on your father's side may all wish to do the same, and if they are not local I will be happy to refer them to genetic counselors in their local areas."

Tearfully, Bella says, "Thank you Shelly, that's very kind. What is it that my brother needs to know? I mean, I get it about the breast and ovarian cancer risks, but why does my brother need to be concerned? Or my son, for that matter?"

"Another good question. While certainly your brother is never going to develop ovarian cancer," Shelly pointed out with a small giggle to lighten the mood a bit, "men can have breast cancer. It is much less likely than it would be in you or your sister, but the risk is increased in men with *BRCA2* mutations. Please remember that we don't know that he has a mutation yet, so this is all only relevant if he does. But if he does, then his breast cancer risk is somewhat elevated, to about 6% over the course of his lifetime, and his prostate cancer risk would be elevated as well. There is no special screening he would need to rule out prostate cancer, but he should be carefully and routinely screened starting at age 40. As for his breast cancer risk, at a minimum, he should perform monthly self-breast exams as well as have his doctor perform annual breast exams. But there is not a lot of clinical evidence regarding breast cancer in men, and treatment standards have been extrapolated from the enormous literature and clinical experience in women. These data may not be entirely applicable to men because their hormones are different. For men who are diagnosed with breast cancer, gender differences may affect patient preferences, toxic effects from therapies, and survivorship priorities. But I think we're getting ahead of ourselves. Let's not worry about these things unless your brother is a carrier, okay?"

"Okay, that's fair," Bella says with a tired smile. "But when should my sister be tested? I just don't want her to have to go through what I'm going through."

Shelly smiled back and spoke gently. "There's no right time. It all depends upon if and when she would like to know, and of course what she might consider doing with the information once she has it. Naturally if she's tested and doesn't have the mutation, she will likely feel much relieved. But if she does turn out to be a carrier, she will be facing some of the same decisions that you are. She will need to think about surveillance options for her breast cancer risk, possible mastectomies as well as hormonal options such as Tamoxifen, and certainly having her ovaries and tubes removed would be highly recommended. Although the breast cancer risk is higher than the ovarian cancer risk, we would actually be more concerned for her ovaries, given the lack of good screening tools for ovarian cancer, so likely her physicians will recommend that she have the surgery by the age of 40–45. But there are a few psychological issues to think about too for Amanda." Bella and Jake look quizzical as Shelly continues. "For example, sometimes when siblings of someone with a mutation in a cancer gene have testing and are not carrying that mutation, they have a reaction similar to survivor's guilt. It can be difficult for non-carriers to relate to their carrier siblings, and many feel badly that they were spared when their siblings were not. Conversely, those with mutations are probably happy for their non-carrier siblings, but at the same time, possibly a little resentful (even if subconsciously) that they themselves carry the mutation when their siblings do not. Of course not all family members will have these types of reactions, but it's just something to think about and perhaps mention to Amanda before she dives into testing. Or if you're not comfortable bringing this up with her, I would be happy to if she would like to come talk with me. And of course she needs to think through when she might be ready to hear whether she has this mutation. Sometimes we find that people jump into testing because they feel like if the information is available that they should have it. But there are times that are not ideal. For example – maybe someone is young and in college. She would have many other big life issues and decisions going on before the knowledge would be necessary for medical management decisions. So it wouldn't necessarily be the best time to pile this information on, psychologically. Likewise, if someone is just having a baby, just lost a job, or is going through a divorce, it can be very difficult to process having a gene mutation as well. Timing is important. Of course there is every bit as much of a chance that Amanda will test negative as that she will test positive, but we can't know ahead of time which it will be. And once she knows, she can't not know, so if she thinks it might be any kind of issue for her, now might not be the best time. But it certainly sounds like you have a very supportive family, and perhaps that's all she needs." Shelly pauses. "What other questions can I answer for you?"

Bella started. "This all makes a lot of sense to me and I hope it will to Amanda as well. I just feel like it's all a little too much right now. Amanda is freaked out by my diagnosis and I hate for her to think that sometime soon she's going to go through it too. Or that she's going to need to have her ovaries out. But I guess if we go through it together maybe it's not so bad."

"That's the spirit," Jake said sarcastically, with no enthusiasm at all.

"What I'm hearing, Jake," Shelly started, "is some fear on your part, am I right?"

"Your damn right I'm scared. My wife is fighting for her life and I just can't worry about Amanda too. We all love her, and I'm glad she's there for Bella, but I have my wife and kids to think about. I just can't take this on too. It's all too much."

"As overwhelming as this feels right now, please remember that there is nothing that needs to be done at this moment. Bella is being well cared for by her oncologist, her surgeon, and her social worker. Amanda is a separate story. You're right – she's not your problem. She is a grown woman who will make her own decisions regarding whether and when to have genetic testing and what to do with the information if and when she has it. No one is asking you to take that on too. You said it best – your job is only to be there for your wife and kids, which you are doing in a very big way right now. No one is asking more of you, right Bella?"

Bella nods and takes Jakes hand in hers. "No baby, I'm not." She looks at Shelly and says "he's my rock. Couldn't do anything without him." She smiles and gives Jake a reassuring smile.

"I can tell!" Shelly says. "Don't expect too much of yourselves right now. The integration of this information can take some time. You need time and space to process it and reprocess it, and come to a 'new normal' in your lives. But you will. And there are support groups if you need them. And social workers on staff who are trained to help people just like you to figure out strategic approaches for managing the complex web of uncertainty that can sometimes challenge people for a lifetime. But that probably sounds worse than it is. You will figure this out. And we are all here to help. Genetic counselors like me are particularly good at helping families manage emotionally challenging risk-related uncertainty. Please don't ever hesitate to call me with questions or concerns or just to talk. Okay? Okay Jake?"

Bella and Jake thank Shelly for all her help and promise to call if they need further assistance and leave the clinic hand in hand. Shelly heads back to her office feeling equal parts satisfied that she helped this lovely couple and sad to have had to give them life-altering news. She knows that she has given them empowering information that will allow Bella to protect herself from a future cancer diagnosis and perhaps protect her family members as well. All in a good day's work!

Pediatric Cancer Complexities

Introduction

Patrick is a 28-year-old male of European descent with a personal history of unilateral retinoblastoma of the right eye diagnosed in childhood. He and his parents had been referred to genetics clinic in the past but had chosen not to follow through in making an appointment. His older sister, Rebecca, is now engaged and has asked him to reconsider pursuing the genetic testing given the potential implications for her and the family as well as for Patrick himself. Although he would prefer not to do this, Patrick contacts the genetic counselor who his doctor has recommended. He completes a family history questionnaire and sets up the appointment for a few weeks from his initial contact with the clinic.

As the date for his genetic counseling appointment approaches, Patrick has conflicting thoughts and emotions. On one hand, he is curious whether his cancer diagnosis was hereditary and something that he could pass on to his future children. On the other hand, he is terrified and does not even want to think about this. He has moved past having cancer as a child, has put his past to rest in his mind, and prefers to avoid thinking any more about it.

Pre-test Genetic Counseling

Today, Patrick comes to the genetics clinic alone. He is anxious about the appointment and reluctant to talk about his personal and family history. During the first few minutes of the appointment, the genetic counselor, Erica, has recognized Patrick's hesitation, and she makes a few attempts to put him at ease. They contract about the plan for their session together. She elicits his primary fears about the appointment and gets to the heart of the information that he is most frightened to hear: that he harbors a disease-causing gene change or mutation in the retinoblastoma gene called RB1. He is quiet for a moment and then shares that he doesn't really know what it would mean to test positive. Erica validates his concern and shares how they will cover that information in detail today. She reassures him that he will leave today with his questions answered and that he does not have to have the blood draw for the actual testing today. This gives him some relief and allows him to keep an open mind as they continue.

Patrick has no family history of retinoblastoma and is the only person to have a diagnosis of any type of cancer other than his maternal grandmother, who was diagnosed with a cancer of unknown primary origin at age 50 and died soon after. His mother does not like to discuss this given how much she, her father, and her siblings struggled while watching the matriarch of the family in pain and suffering. His mother had a preventative gynecologic surgery at a relatively young age and Patrick assumes that this was related to his grandmother's personal history.

Table 5.2 Heritable and nonheritable forms of retinoblastoma

Feature	Nonheritable	Heritable
Retinoblastoma tumor	Unilateral	Usually bilateral or multifocal
Family history	None	~20% of cases
Average age at diagnosis	~2 years	<1 year
Increased risk of second primary tumors	No	Osteosarcoma, soft tissue sarcomas, melanoma, others
RB1 mutations found	In tumors only (somatic)	In germline and in tumors

Source: American Society of Clinical Oncology 2004, Abramson & Frank, 1998, Kleinerman, Yu, Little, et al., 2012

The genetic counselor makes a recommendation for Patrick's mother to pursue individualized genetic counseling to explore this further. Patrick knows that his mother was proud of him for making today's appointment, and he thinks that he can talk with his mom about the recommendation for her to see a counselor now that he is going through the process himself.

Following the review of his family history, the focus returns to Patrick's personal history. Given that Patrick was diagnosed with one tumor in one eye and at 16 months of age, Erica provides a risk assessment which is surprising and somewhat reassuring to him. His chance of having a mutation in the RB1 gene is not nearly as high as he suspected it to be! However, there are many possibilities, and he needs to be tested in order to truly determine his status and risk for other types of cancer. With the approximate 15% chance of having a germline RB1 mutation, Patrick now feels better equipped to hear the rest of the information and participate in the discussion more than he did at the start of the session (Lohmann, Gerick, Brandt, et al., 1997; Lohmann & Gallie, 2017; Temming, Viehmann, Biewald, & Lohmann, 2013). They review the differences between heritable and nonheritable forms of retinoblastoma as currently understood (summarized in Table 5.2). Patrick has heard about the increased risk to develop cancers outside of the eye but is curious about what is known and ready to acquire more knowledge on this topic. He also admits to feeling very guilty since he has not maintained contact with his treating physicians the past few years and has not been screening for these secondary tumors recently. He has preferred to defer doing this until undergoing genetic testing. Erica again validates his underlying fears and shares how she will address the screening recommendations in their discussion today.

Before Erica delves into the primary and secondary tumor risks associated with RB1 mutations, she addresses the categories of test results. Patrick learns a lot from the discussion as he becomes more comfortable. He hears about the types of test results (summarized in Table 5.3), including what low-level mosaicism means (some of the cells of his body may carry one copy of the RB1 gene mutation, while most of his cells may not carry it). For a brief moment, he almost wishes for a positive mosaic result so that the likelihood for his sister Rebecca (and therefore her future children) to share the mutation would be incredibly low (Carlson & Desnick,

Table 5.3 Summary of the interpretation of RB1 test results

Type of *RB1* test result	Possible interpretation	Recommendations/options
Positive[a]	Pathogenic, deleterious mutation identified = thought to be causative of disease	Cancer screening and risk reduction strategies Predictive testing for family members Family planning options
Variant of uncertain significance[a]	Pathogenic, polymorphism, *or* no significance	Segregation and functional studies may be performed on a new blood sample Medical management based on history No testing available for family members (with the exception of segregation studies on a research basis)
Negative (no variant or mutation identified)	*For patients with bilateral or multifocal RB* = uninformative (i.e., may be an occult mutation or a different gene involved) *For patients with unifocal unilateral RB* = reduces likelihood of a mutation (i.e., may be sporadic) *For unaffected relatives of a proband with an RB1 mutation* = considered "true" negative	Medical management based on personal history No testing available for family members

Source: Carlson & Desnick, 1979; Rushlow et al., 2009; Sippel et al., 1998
[a]Mosaicism (i.e., some of the cells of the body carry one copy of the RB1 gene mutation, while others cells do not carry it) is possible for both positive and uncertain results

1979; Rushlow, Piovesan, Zhang, et al., 2009; Sippel, Fraioli, Smith, et al., 1998). But he is still hoping for a negative result and is reassured given that his chances for a negative result are high (approximately 85%) (Lohmann & Gallie, 2017).

As Erica reviews the meaning of uncertain results, called variations of uncertain significance, Patrick's anxiety creeps up again. He does not want to have to face potential future cancer risks and the recommended screening – all without a positive result to confirm the risks or to support the need for the screening. Patrick begins to relax once again as the possibility for uncertain results is put into context in terms of being a possibility any time genetic testing is performed, as well as the clarification that this would be a rare result. In addition, variations of uncertain significance may be reclassified with more information and are most often reclassified to be negative results that are not associated with an increased cancer risk (Dimaras et al., 2012; Knudson, 1971; Knudson, 1976; Lohmann & Gallie, 2004; Zhang et al., 2015).

Erica helps Patrick to think in detail about what he would do with the information if he were to test positive (summarized in Table 5.4). As they discuss this further, Patrick begins to feel optimistic in exploring the potential benefits of a positive test

Table 5.4 Potential benefits and uses of positive RBI germline test results

Patients with bilateral or unilateral multifocal RB who test positive for an RB1 mutation:
Confirms the explanation for the diagnosis in the patient
Confirms the type of mutation (e.g., mosaic, etc.) and assists with the recommendation for long-term follow-up and screening for secondary tumors
Allows the identification of the mutation in parents, siblings, children, and extended relatives and allows true negative result for the proband's siblings and children
Provides reproductive options now or in the future for the proband and also any of his/her relatives who are identified to harbor the same *RB1* mutation
Patients with unilateral unifocal RB who test positive for an RB1 mutation:
Provides an explanation for the diagnosis in the proband
Supports current medical management for the risk to the other eye (regular exams under anesthesia until at least 44 months of age)
Guides future medical management for secondary tumors and long-term follow-up
Allows the identification of the mutation in parents, siblings, children, and extended relatives and allows true negative result for the proband's siblings and children
Provides reproductive options now or in the future for the proband and also any of his/her relatives who are identified to harbor the same *RB1* mutation
Unaffected relatives who test positive for an RB1 mutation:
Guides future medical management for secondary tumors and long-term follow-up
Allows the identification of the mutation in other relatives and allows true negative result for their own children
Provides reproductive options for the patient and any of their other relatives who are identified to harbor the same *RB1* mutation

Source: Lohmann & Gallie, 2017

result when thinking of this as a theoretical possibility. He recognizes how a positive result would give his physicians more guidance for his long-term follow-up and give him steps to take. The thought of taking action makes him feel much more empowered than standing still in fear.

Uncertainty Related to Future Cancers in Those Already Diagnosed

As mentioned earlier in their discussion, Patrick has several questions about the secondary tumors associated with germline RB1 mutations. Erica shares the information that is currently known about the tumor types and the associated risks to develop osteosarcomas, soft tissue sarcomas, melanoma, and some other specific cancers. She also reviews how the types of treatments from the past may have contributed to the estimated risks and how the type of RB1 gene test result (e.g., mosaic) may also influence the risk of other cancer types. It is frustrating to Patrick how much uncertainty surrounds these numbers and how these are estimates based on small studies. He would prefer to know exactly when to plan for a second tumor, if at all. Erica validates his concern and admits her own struggles with uncertainty.

At the same time, she offers an alternative perspective to help him to think about this as empowering information which can be used to take action with cancer screening. She also shares the option to meet with a clinical psychologist who works with their team and may help him to compartmentalize this information, whether he were to receive negative, uncertain, or positive results. He finds this suggestion promising and takes the contact information for the psychologist who specializes in working with individuals at risk for cancer.

Options for Cancer Surveillance

Patrick asks Erica to describe the details for screening for the secondary tumor types. She shares how investigation of any signs or symptoms is recommended as well as annual eye examinations, physical examinations, and a complete blood count (CBC). Total body imaging with magnetic resonance imaging (MRI) is under study to determine whether it is specific and sensitive enough for screening for second cancers in individuals who harbor a germline RB1 mutation (Lohmann & Gallie, 2017). After they review this together, Patrick feels fortunate that he is an adult now and able to think about the cancer screening regime as objectively as possible, drawing on his maturity level and life experience to date. While he understands the limitations of screening, he appreciates the potential benefit of catching a new cancer at the earliest stage possible and how this does not have to consume his life going forward. He is able to put the plan for the screening into the big picture and think about what he may want to do to make this easier on himself mentally each time, as well as how he could design the appointments to fit into his schedule. It would not be as big a deal or need to be as daunting a task as he once assumed!

Reproductive Options

When Erica explains the options for future reproduction, Patrick almost jumps up out of his seat! He did not realize how much is available to couples who harbor a germline mutation in many different genes, let alone someone with a predisposition to develop retinoblastoma. The option of preimplantation genetic diagnosis (PGD; discussed in more detail earlier in this chapter) or testing early-stage embryos for an RB1 mutation (if identified in his blood sample) gives him immense relief (Xu, Rosenwaks, Beaverson, et al., 2004). He loves the idea of stopping this and preventing him from passing on the high risk of having bilateral retinoblastoma to his future children. This conversation leaves room for him to think about how he would be able to have many options if he chooses to get married in the future. That seems far away to him now but he knows how close and real this is for his sister.

Concern for Family Members at Risk

Patrick shares how the impetus for him to come today was primarily based on his sister's encouragement. He is aware how she and other family members may benefit from the information obtained from his test results. Erica reviews the autosomal dominant inheritance pattern for germline RB1 mutations but also explains how his mutation would mostly likely have been a de novo mutation and happened by chance early in his development as opposed to having been inherited from his mother or father. He is very motivated to share this information with his sister and with his parents. Patrick wants his mom to stop worrying about him and let go of the past. He knows how his dad has also carried fears about Patrick's health although he has been much quieter about them. Patrick hopes that even if he tests positive, this will help his family to be tested and find out their status one way or the other. He is reassured that most of them would be "true negatives;" his parents and sister would not likely harbor an RB1 mutation even if he does.

At the end of the pre-test counseling session, Patrick feels as ready as possible to proceed with having his blood sample drawn. He has asked all of the questions that he can think of at this time and has gathered quite a bit of information. He has been provided with a few options and is aware of the plan to meet with Erica as well as a physician to receive his test results in person. He has scheduled his results disclosure appointment to be later this spring, on a date when he will be visiting his family the following weekend.

He provides his written consent for the testing and has his blood drawn. Erica encourages him to contact her with any questions in the interim period. She also reminds him that he is welcome to make an appointment with the psychologist if he chooses to, now or after receiving his test results. He is genuinely grateful for Erica's time and expertise and thanks her.

Results Disclosure

The day arrives for Patrick's follow-up genetic counseling appointment to receive his results. He slept well and feels ready for what may come his way.

Erica immediately smiles when greeting him in the reception area. "I have good news for you," she says. He sighs and walks with her to her office. "Your results are negative!" A sense of relief washes over Patrick from head to toe. She gives him a few moments to respond and asks what he is thinking. Patrick articulates his immense relief and then asks to see the report. They review the results in detail, including the remaining residual risk for the possibility of very low-level mosaicism, given that there was no tumor tissue available and only DNA from his blood sample was tested. A less than 1% risk for this is music to his ears (Lohmann & Gallie, 2017; Rushlow, Mol, Kennett, et al., 2013; Thériault, Dimaras, Gallie, & Corson, 2014). He is aware of the small possibility for his future children, but now he can look his parents and sister in the eye this weekend and share the wonderful news – no testing is required for them and they are back to general population risk! Patrick will reconnect with his treating physician to share these results and set up annual eye examinations. He will stay in touch with Erica for any questions in the future and prior to planning his family. After more of a discussion with Erica and an attending physician, Patrick has one remaining question, which is more for himself than anyone else–"why did I wait so long to come here?"

Conclusions

Using two detailed case examples, we have illustrated the complicated issues surrounding genetic counseling and genetic testing for adult and pediatric cancer families. While providing genetic testing is an important component of medical care, there are other elements arguably more critical to patients with personal and family histories of cancer (Resta, 2017). These may include an intense exploration of the psychological and personal facets of why people may choose to have testing as well as which tests they choose to have. Genetic counselors are specifically trained to support and work with patients whether they have testing or not, when testing is postponed due to lack of insurance, indecision, or lack of supporting family documentation, when testing is irrelevant, or when testing was done in the past and they need help in adapting to their new medical and emotional status. It is vital to explore what the personal and family histories have meant for the patient's life, what resources he or she might need, who else in the family might be affected, and how they might or might not be supportive of each other, as well as the medical, economic, and social impacts of genetic disease. Providing genetic testing to patients and their physicians is important, certainly, but providing patients with the tools they need to understand the results or even decide whether they would like to have the results in the first place and how they would negotiate them into their lives is far more important and requires skill and finesse.

References

American Society of Clinical Oncology. (2004). ASCO slide library. http://boa.asco.org/virtual-meeting-and-oncology-slide-library

Abramson, D. A., & Frank, C. M. (1998). Second nonocular tumors in survivors of bilateral retinoblastoma. *Ophthalmology*, *105*(4), 573–580.

Buys, S. S., Partridge, E., Black, A., Johnson, C., Lamerato, L., Isaacs, C., … Reding, D. (2011). Effect of screening on ovarian cancer mortality in the Prostate, Lung, Colorectal, and Ovarian (PLCO) cancer randomized screening trial. *Journal of Clinical Oncology*, *29*(15 suppl), 5001.

Carlson, E. A., & Desnick, R. J. (1979). Mutational mosaicism and genetic counseling in retinoblastoma. *American Journal of Medical Genetics*, *4*, 365–381.

Chen, S., & Parmigiani, G. (2007). Meta-analysis of BRCA1 and BRCA2 penetrance. *Journal of Clinical Oncology*, *25*(11), 1329–1333.

Couch, F. J., Shimelis, H., Hu, C., Hart, S. N., Polley, E. C., & Na, J. (2017). Associations between cancer predisposition testing panel genes and breast cancer. *JAMA 3*(9), 1190–1196.

Dimaras, H., Kimani, K., Dimba, E. A. O., Gronsdahl, P., White, A., Chan, H. S. L., Gallie, B. L. (2012). Retinoblastoma. *The Lancet 379*(9824):1436–1446.

Kleinerman, R. A., Yu, C. L., Little, M. P., Li, Y., Abramson, D., Seddon, J., … Tucker, M. A. (2012). Variation of second cancer by family history among long-term survivors. *Journal of Clinical Oncology, 30*, 950–957.

Knudson, A. G. (1971). Mutation and cancer: Statistical study of retinoblastoma. *Proceedings of National Science, 68*, 820–823.

Knudson, A. G. (1976). Genetics and the etiology of childhood cancer. *Pediatric Research, 10*(5), 513–517.

Kuchenbaecker, K. B., Hopper, J. L., Barnes, D. R., Phillips, K., Mooij, T. M., Roos-Blom, M., … Jervis, S. (2017). Risks of breast, ovarian, and contralateral breast cancer for *BRCA1* and *BRCA2* mutation carriers. *JAMA, 317*(23), 2402–2416.

Lee, V. C. Y., Chow, J. F. C., Yeung, W. S. B., & Ho, P. C. (2017). Preimplantation genetic diagnosis for monogenic diseases. *Best Practice & Research. Clinical Obstetrics & Gynaecology, 44*, 68–75. *S1521-6934(17)30055-X.*

Lohmann, D., Gerick, M., Brandt, B., Oelschläger, U., Lorenz, B., Passarge, E., … Horsthemke, B. (1997). Constitutional *RB1* gene mutations in patients with isolated unilateral retinoblastoma. *American Journal of Human Genetics, 61*(2), 282–294.

Lohmann, D. R., & Gallie, B. L. (2017). Retinoblastoma. *Gene Reviews.* Retrieved from http://www.ncbi.nlm.nih.gov/bookshelf/br.fcgi?book=gene&part=retinoblastoma

Lohmann, D. R., & Gallie, B. L. (2004). Retinoblastoma: Revisiting the model prototype of inherited cancer. *American Journal of Medical Genetics, 129C*, 23–28.

Mavaddat, N., Peock, S., Frost, D., Ellis, S., Platte, R., Fineberg, E., … Evans, D. G. (2013). Cancer risks for BRCA1 and BRCA2 mutation carriers: Results from prospective analysis of EMBRACE. *Journal of the National Cancer Institute, 105*(11), 812–822.

Mersch, J., Jackson, M. A., Park, M., Nebgen, D., Peterson, S. K., & Singletary, C. (2015). Cancers associated with BRCA1 and BRCA2 mutations other than breast and ovarian. *Cancer, 121*, 269–275.

Myriad Genetic Laboratories. (2017). Retrieved 6/9/17 https://myriad-web.s3.amazonaws.com/myriad.com/pdf/Myriad-Corporate-Presentation.pdf

Offit, K., Kohut, K., Clagett, B., Wadsworth, E. A., Lafaro, K. J., Cummings, S., … White, M. (2006). Cancer genetic testing and assisted reproduction. *Journal of Clinical Oncology, 24*(29), 4775–4782.

Rahman, N., Seal, S., Thompson, D., Kelly, P., Renwick, A., Elliott, A., … Reid, S. (2007). PALB2, which encodes a BRCA2-interacting protein, is a breast cancer susceptibility gene. *Nature Genetics, 39*(2), 165–167.

Renwick, A., Thompson, D., Seal, S., Kelly, P., Chagtai, T., Ahmed, M., … North, B. (2006). ATM mutations that cause ataxia-telangiectasia are breast cancer susceptibility alleles. *Nature Genetics, 38*(8), 873–875.

Resta, R. (2017). Genetic Counseling ≠ Genetic Testing. Retrieved from *The DNA Exchange*, 7/5/17.

Rushlow, D., Mol, B. M., Kennett, J. Y., Yee, S., Pajovic, S., Thériault, B. L., … Prigoda-Lee, N. L. (2013). Characterization of retinoblastomas without *RB1* mutations: Genomic, gene expression, and clinical studies. *The Lancet Oncology, 14*(4), 327–334.

Rushlow, D., Piovesan, B., Zhang, K., Prigoda-Lee, N. L., Marchong, M. N., Clark, R. D., … Gallie, B. L. (2009). Detection of mosaic *RB1* mutations in families with retinoblastoma. *Human Mutation, 30*, 842–851.

Sagi, M., Weinberg, N., Eilat, A., Aizenman, E., Werner, M., Girsh, E., … Siminovsky, Y. (2009). Preimplantation genetic diagnosis for BRCA1/2–a novel clinical experience. *Prenatal Diagnosis, 29*(5), 508–513.

Schrader, K. A., Cheng, D. T., Joseph, V., Prasad, M., Walsh, M., Zehir, A., … Ni, A. (2016). Germline variants in targeted tumor sequencing using matched normal DNA. *JAMA Oncology, 2*(1), 104–111.

Sippel, K. C., Fraioli, R. E., Smith, G. D., Schalkoff, M. E., Sutherland, J., Gallie, B. L., … Dryja, T. P. (1998). Frequency of somatic and germ-line mosaicism in retinoblastoma: Implications for genetic counseling. *American Journal of Human Genetics, 62*, 610–619.

Temming, P., Viehmann, A., Biewald, E., & Lohmann, D. R. (2013). Sporadic unilateral retinoblastoma or first sign of bilateral disease? *British Journal of Opthalmology, 97*, 475–480.

Thériault, B. L., Dimaras, H., Gallie, B. L., & Corson, T. W. (2014). The genomic landscape of retinoblastoma: A review. *Clinical & Experimental Ophthalmology, 42*, 33–52.

Tung, N., Domchek, S. M., Stadler, Z., Nathanson, K. L., Couch, F., Garber, J. E., … Offit, K. (2016). Counselling framework for moderate-penetrance cancer-susceptibility mutations. *Nature Reviews Clinical Oncology, 13*(9), 581–588.

Walsh, T., Casadei, S., Lee, M. K., Pennil, C. C., Nord, A. S., Thornton, A. M., … Roeb, W. (2011). Mutations in 12 genes for inherited ovarian, fallopian tube, and peritoneal carcinoma identified by massively parallel sequencing. *Proceedings of the National Academy of Sciences of the United States of America, 108*(44), 18032–18037.

Walsh, T., & King, M. C. (2007). Ten genes for inherited breast cancer. *Cancer Cell, 11*(2), 103–105.

Xu, K., Rosenwaks, Z., Beaverson, K., Cholst, I., Veeck, L., & Abramson, D. H. (2004). Preimplantation genetic diagnosis for retinoblastoma: The first reported Liveborn. *American Journal of Ophthalmology, 137*(1), 18–23.

Zhang, J., Walsh, M. F., Wu, G., Edmonson, M. N., Gruber, T. A., Easton, J., … Hedges, D. (2015). Germline mutations in predisposition genes in pediatric cancer. *The New England Journal of Medicine, 373*(24), 2336–2346.

Chapter 6
Quality of Life Among Patients With Tongue Cancer: Primary Closure Versus Free Flap Reconstruction

Feras Al Halabi

Introduction

Oral cancers have the 7th and 13th highest incidence in the United States and Canada, respectively (Chong, 2005). Oral squamous cell carcinoma accounts for 24% of all head and neck cancers and often arises due to a combination of genetic alterations and continuous exposure to environmental agents such as tobacco and alcohol (Carvalho, Nishimoto, Califano, & Kowalski, 2004). Among European and North American populations, the tongue is the most common site for intraoral cancer, amounting to almost half of all oral cancers (Warnakulasuriya, 2009). It was estimated that in 2010, 10,990 new cases were diagnosed and 1990 patients had died of tongue cancer in the United States (Siegel, Naishadham, & Jemal, 2013). Typically, these aggressive lesions affect men aged 60–80 but can occur in the very young as well. Recently, tongue cancer has shown a fivefold increase in younger adults aged 20–44 years and a twofold increase in older adults (Shiboski, Schmidt, & Jordan, 2005). Tongue cancer is particularly dangerous because of a high risk of spreading to nearby lymph nodes and therefore has major implications for future well-being and quality of life among cancer survivors (Chong, 2005). More importantly, the tongue is one of the most difficult structures of the oral cavity to reconstruct because of its central role in articulation, deglutition, and airway protection (Engel, 2010).

F. Al Halabi (✉)
Faculty of Dentistry, McGill University, Montreal, QC, Canada
e-mail: feras.alhalabi@mail.mcgill.ca

T. R. Fitzpatrick (ed.), *Quality of Life Among Cancer Survivors*,
https://doi.org/10.1007/978-3-319-75223-5_6

Anatomy

The tongue lacks an internal skeletal structure, has a muscular architecture of three-dimensional orthogonal muscles, and maintains a constant volume as it deforms during function, allowing for highly complex and virtually infinite shapes to be achieved (Reichard, Stone, & Woo, 2012). The tongue is composed of two main muscle groups: the intrinsic and extrinsic muscles. The intrinsic muscles are all confined within the body of the tongue and are longitudinal with both superior and inferior components, transverse and vertical (Hamlet, Mathog, Patterson, & Fleming, 1990). These muscles serve mainly to deform the tongue for proper mastication, deglutition, and phonation. The four extrinsic muscles of the tongue, which originate outside of the tongue body, are the genioglossus, hyoglossus, styloglossus, and palatoglossus muscles. These muscles function to protrude, depress, and elevate the tongue, respectively (Hamlet et al., 1990). The finely coordinated contraction of the intrinsic and extrinsic muscles allows for the organ to carry out highly complex movements of speech, mastication, and swallowing (Hamlet et al., 1990; Suarez-Cunqueiro et al., 2008). Loss of integrity in any of these muscles severely impairs speech quality and swallowing (Suarez-Cunqueiro et al., 2008).

Tumors can involve the oral tongue, the base of tongue, or both; the anatomical point of separation is the circumvallate papillae. The site of most tongue cancers is the anterior two-thirds of the lateral border or the ventral surface (Chong, 2005). Adequate oncologic control of squamous cell carcinoma often necessitates aggressive surgical resection to ensure clear margins and minimize the risk of recurrence. Whereas 1 cm is generally considered adequate for most squamous cell carcinomas, for tongue cancer, it has been suggested that margins should be 1.5–2 cm given the high chance for local or regional recurrence (Chong, 2005). Glossectomy is often carried out as a therapeutic means to eradicate tongue malignancies (Spiro & Strong, 1974). The highly complex coordination of different muscles of the tongue produces the necessary precise movements for proper speech, mastication, and deglutition (Urken, 2003; Urken, Moscoso, Lawson, & Biller, 1994). How a patient adapts after the removal of tongue tissue might be dependent on the type of closure/reconstruction that is performed; however, there remains controversy regarding which of these specific procedures offers the patient the best functional outcomes. The importance of this question has led to the production of many articles that have clearly discussed the effect of oncologic ablative surgery for tongue squamous cell carcinoma and the significant comorbidity, specifically, due to the effects on speech and swallowing (Hara, Gellrich, Duker, Schön, Fakler, et al., 2003; Stelzle, Knipfer, Schuster, & Bocklet, 2013; Suarez-Cunqueiro et al., 2008; Urken et al., 1994). This in turn, plays a major role in the quality of life of patients post glossectomy (Hartl et al., 2009; Radford, Woods, & Lowe, 2004).

Quality of Life

The tongue is the key structure for pronunciation, sustenance, and communication. Patients suffering from tongue malignancies have significantly lower intelligibility scores than control patients, even before surgical intervention (Stelzle et al., 2013). Further impairment occurs after surgical rehabilitation and is closely related to tumor localization and the volume of resection which is guided by the tumor size (Borggreven et al., 2005; Matsui, Ohno, Yamashita, & Takahashi, 2007; Stelzle et al., 2013; Sun, Weng, Li, Wang, & Zhang, 2007). Loss of tongue mass and motor control, which occurs during glossectomy, creates challenges in reaching the palate and elevating the tongue tip during speech (Chuanjun, 2002; Reichard et al., 2012; Sun et al., 2007). Patients whose speech and swallowing are affected following treatment and surgery for tongue cancer may experience difficulties in communication as speaking may be affected together with health and nutrition issues resulting in increased isolation, possible depression, and loneliness. The surgical treatment of tongue cancer, with or without reconstruction and/or radiotherapy, leads to different levels of voice, speech, and deglutition disorders. Evaluating the quality of life related to these swallowing alterations is important to further our knowledge about the impact of such alterations from the patient's point of view (Costa Bandeira et al., 2008, p. 183). These authors studied the quality of life related to swallowing in patients treated for tongue cancer. Findings revealed that the aspects related to how to deal with deglutition problems, time taken for meal consumption, pleasure in eating, chewing problems, food sticking in the throat and mouth, choking, and the knowledge of feeding restrictions, which were evaluated by different domains of SWAL-QOL, were factors that contributed to a negative impact for patients with advanced-stage tumors who underwent radiotherapy (Costa Bandeira et al., 2008, p. 183).

Swallowing is an automatically regulated process until trauma occurs (Dodds, Logemann, & Stewart, 1990). After surgical intervention, patients show a significant decline in swallowing ability, with a level of dysfunction closely related to tumor stage, site, and extent of its excision within the oral cavity (Hsiao, Leu, & Lin, 2002; Logemann et al., 1993; Nicoletti, Soutar, Jackson, Wrench, & Robertson, 2004; O'Connell et al., 2008; Pauloski et al., 1993). Reconstructive treatments for oral cavity cancers involving the tongue are aimed at preserving the patient's ability to swallow and speak whenever possible (Engel, 2010). However, reconstruction following tongue cancer resection remains one of the most challenging problems in head and neck oncology (Engel, 2010). The principles of reconstruction traditionally follow a reconstructive ladder; small glossectomy defects may be closed by primary closure, healing by secondary intention, or with the use of skin grafts, while greater resections necessitate reconstructions with local, pedicled, or free flaps (Bokhari & Wang, 2007; Urken et al., 1994). The choice of reconstruction selected after tongue cancer resection plays a major role in the ultimate speech and swallowing abilities of the patient (Hsiao et al., 2002; Khariwala et al., 2007; Logemann et al., 1993; Nicoletti, Soutar, Jackson, Wrench, & Robertson, 2004; O'Connell et al., 2008; Pauloski et al., 1993, 2004; Su, 2003). Although, postoperative function is influenced by multiple factors, such as location, other structures in the area that are resected, and radiation, it is clear that restoration of mobility and bulk of the tongue is essential to achieving optimal outcomes (Hsiao et al., 2002; Hsiao, Leu, Chang, & Lee, 2003; Hsiao, Leu, & Lin, 2003). Quality of life during postoperative recovery will be greatly impacted by the success of the reconstruction surgery and the individual's ability to adjust and cope with the changes in speech and swallowing.

Techniques

Tongue reconstruction to restore its functionality after resection has been greatly advanced by the predictable use of microvascular free flap techniques (Khariwala et al., 2007). Although there is a clearer understanding on the technique to employ when dealing with the extremes of defects, there is a lack of consensus among clinicians as to the best method of reconstruction for a medium-sized defect (hemiglossectomy defect). There are advocates for both primary closure and flap reconstruction with differences in outcomes based on limited retrospective data (Bressmann, Ackloo, Heng, & Irish, 2007; Chuanjun, 2002; Hsiao et al., 2003; McConnel et al., 1998). There are numerous studies reporting on the use of a variety of free flaps to reconstruct partial or hemiglossectomy defects; however, there is not enough data comparing speech, swallow, and quality of life outcomes postsurgery (de Vicente, de Villalaín, Torre, & Peña, 2008; Matsui et al., 2007; Matsui, Shirota, Yamashita, & Ohno, 2009; Seikaly et al., 2003; Su, 2003; Sun et al., 2007). This review presents the available evidence for primary closure or free flap reconstruction for partial or hemiglossectomy defects. We also present the determinants and outcome measures used in the present literature to evaluate the functional outcome of speech and swallowing after surgical rehabilitation.

Functional Outcomes of Glossectomy, Reconstruction, and Quality of Life

Previous studies have concentrated their evaluations on speech and swallowing, factors which are most negatively affected by surgical ablation (Suarez-Cunqueiro et al., 2008). These are also the factors that patients usually identify as having a large effect on their quality of life (Dwivedi, Kazi, Agrawal, & Nutting, 2009; List et al., 2000). A number of determinants have been identified to affect the functional outcomes after glossectomy and surgical rehabilitation (Matsui et al., 2007, 2009; Reichard et al., 2012; Stelzle et al., 2013; Sun et al., 2007).

Speech: Determinants of Functional Outcome

Tumor site, sizes including volume of resection, mobility of the remaining native tongue, method of reconstruction, and postoperative radiotherapy have all been shown to determine postoperative articulation intelligibility after glossectomy. A number of studies have discussed the relationship between speech and tumor site or location (Matsui et al., 2007; McConnel et al., 1998; Pauloski et al., 2004; Pauloski, Logemann, & Rademaker, 1994; Seikaly et al., 2003; Stelzle et al., 2013; Sun et al., 2007). Most studies showed that independent of the method of reconstruction, patients who underwent resection of the anterior portion of the oral tongue had significantly lower intelligibility scores than those who had resection of the middle or posterior third of the oral tongue (Matsui et al., 2007; Sun et al., 2007). Matsui et al. analyzed the intelligibility of 126 patients classified into 3 groups based on the site of tongue resection. Although the type of flap used had no effect on the functional outcome, they concluded that low speech intelligibility scores were recorded when the flap directly contributed to pronunciation in the anterior, lateral, and combined anterolateral resection groups (Matsui et al., 2009). Similarly, Sun et al. showed that patients with preservation of the tongue tip and floor of the mouth showed significantly less decline in intelligibility than those with resection of these sites (Sun et al., 2007). On the other hand, resection of the tongue base did not significantly affect articulation. They concluded that the attempt to preserve the anterior third of the tongue, specifically the tip, and floor of the mouth as much as possible has positive results on speech outcome (Sun et al., 2007).

It is well established that the greater the extent of tongue resection, the poorer the functional outcome (Colangelo, Logemann, & Rademaker, 2000; Matsui et al., 2007; Pauloski et al., 1998; Pauloski et al., 2004; Rieger, 2007; Stelzle et al., 2013; Sun et al., 2007). Patients with advanced primary tumors did significantly worse than patients with smaller tumors in the assessments before and after treatment, concerning communicative suitability, intelligibility, articulation, and consonant errors (Borggreven et al., 2005). Sun et al. showed that patients with T3 tumors had significantly greater decline in intelligibility than the T1 group (Sun et al., 2007). Similarly, Stelzle et al. showed that speech intelligibility in patients with T1 tumors was significantly higher than in patients with larger T2 or T4 tumors. At 12 months postoperatively, the volume of resection was closely related to the functional outcome independently of tumor stage (Stelzle et al., 2013). Hence, patients with larger tongue resection volumes consistently had lower intelligibility scores (Pauloski et al., 1998). Most studies used tumor stage as a mean of identifying tumor size (Colangelo et al., 2000; Matsui et al., 2007; Pauloski et al., 1998, 2004; Rieger, 2007; Stelzle et al., 2013; Sun et al., 2007). Although tumor stage has not explicitly been shown to affect functional outcome, tumor size presents a reliable determinant of speech outcomes. Current research has yet to provide evidence on the percentage of tongue resection or tumor stage that indicates free flap reconstruction to produce a better functional outcome.

Various studies have compared speech outcomes in patients based on the method of reconstruction (Chuanjun, 2002; de Vicente et al., 2008; Hsiao et al., 2002; Matsui et al., 2007; McConnel et al., 1998; Nicoletti et al., 2004; Sun et al., 2007; Thankappan et al., 2011). Conflicting results have been reported on the postoperative motion of the tongue with different techniques for closure selected, whether primary closure or flap reconstruction. Hsiao et al. and Chuanjun et al. found poorer intelligibility and articulation when comparing a radial forearm free flap (RFFF) reconstruction of hemiglossectomy to primary closure (Chuanjun, 2002; Hsiao et al., 2002). Others studying the difference between free flaps found no significant difference in speech outcomes between RFFF and reconstruction with adjacent tongue dorsal flap (Sun et al., 2007), anterolateral thigh flap (ALTF) (de Vicente et al., 2008), rectus abdominis myocutaneous flap (RAMCF), or pectoralis major musculocutaneous flap (PMF) (Matsui et al., 2007). Some data has suggested that a more thin pliable flap such as the RFFF reconstruction resulted in higher intelligibility in certain articulatory sites and modes compared to RAMCF reconstruction of lateral oral tongue defects (Matsui et al., 2009).

Regardless of the method of reconstruction used, it is commonly agreed that mixed modality treatment involving postoperative radiotherapy is associated with poor speech outcomes (Matsui et al., 2007; Nicoletti, Soutar, Jackson, Wrench, Robertson, & Robertson, 2004; Pauloski et al., 1994; Shin, Koh, Kim, Jeong, & Ahn, 2012; Suarez-Cunqueiro et al., 2008; Thankappan et al., 2011; Zuydam, Lowe, Brown, Vaughan, & Rogers, 2005). Shin et al. found that postoperative radiotherapy negatively influenced speech and swallowing in patients with partial glossectomy and RFFF reconstruction (Shin et al., 2012). Patients who were treated by surgery and postoperative radiotherapy had significantly worse speech repetition rates than those treated by surgery only (Shin et al., 2012). Other retrospective studies found that patients who had postoperative radiotherapy had restricted diet and tongue mobility and poorer subjective and objective speech outcomes (Matsui et al., 2007; Thankappan et al., 2011). Although there was no difference in tongue mobility, radiotherapy may have induced more tongue shrinkage than expected preoperatively and thus resulted in a decrease in coordinated tongue movement (Shin et al., 2012; Thankappan et al., 2011). Yun et al. reported that unexpected volume loss of reconstructed tongue tissue can lead to a decreased ability to swallow or speak intelligibly (Yun et al., 2010).

Speech: Assessment Methods

When assessing speech, most studies used perceptual, acoustic, and subjective methods. In perceptual evaluation, recorded speech from the patient under standardized conditions is presented to one or many blinded listeners. The listeners then transcribe the patients' speech for different functional parameters and rate it. The most commonly assessed speech parameters include speech intelligibility, communicative understandability, speech acceptability, articulation, reading time, type of speech errors, and diadochokinetic rate (de Vicente et al., 2008; Hsiao et al., 2002; Hsiao, Leu, & Lin, 2003; Loewen, Boliek, Harris, & Seikaly, 2010; Matsui et al., 2009; Rieger, Zalmanowitz, & Wolfaardt, 2006; Shin et al., 2012; Sun et al., 2007; Thankappan et al., 2011; Uwiera, Seikaly, Rieger, Chau, & Harris, 2004; Yun et al., 2010).

Speech intelligibility is the most common evaluated parameter and includes intelligibility of consonants, vowels, and syllables, as well as words, sentences, and conversations (Bressmann, Sader, Whitehill, & Samman, 2004; Loewen et al., 2010; Matsui et al., 2007; Stelzle et al., 2013; Uwiera et al., 2004). A number of studies graded intelligibility on a scale of 1–7 based on the number of errors the patient produces (de Vicente et al., 2008; Hsiao et al., 2002; Hsiao, Leu, & Lin, 2003; Rieger, 2007; Uwiera et al., 2004). The intelligibility scale they used relied on the number of errors the patient produces, while the articulation scale measured the patient's extent of dysarthria or mispronunciation (Hsiao et al., 2002; Hsiao, Leu, & Lin, 2003). Articulation is usually evaluated by the intelligibility test, because speech is a social tool whose most significant measurement should be how well it is understood (Michi, 2003). Analysis on the basis of articulatory mode and site can determine the sources of speech disorders, regardless of the language in which the test is carried out (Michiwaki, Schmelzeisen, Hacki, & Michi, 1992). The manner by which the tongue interacts with other structures in the oral cavity determines the articulatory mode. The articulatory mode of glossal sounds is composed of seven groups including plosives, fricatives, affricatives, grids, nasals, vowels, and semivowels. Evaluating errors in speech based on articulatory site and mode allows an evaluator to draw conclusions on the effect of reconstruction on speech based on the site and size of resection. In addition, analysis of tongue mobility and effect of volume of resection on speech is carried out by understanding deficits in articulation based on articulatory site and mode.

Measurement of diadochokinetic (DDK) rate is a test used by speech-language pathologists (SLP) to assess, diagnose, and treat speech malfunctions (Gadesmann & Miller, 2008). It is also known as the Fletcher Time-by-Count Test of Diadochokinetic Syllable Rate. DDK rate measures how quickly a person can accurately repeat a series of rapid, alternating phonetic sounds. These sounds, called tokens, are designed to test different parts of the mouth, tongue, and soft palate in the back of the throat. The tokens contain one, two, or three syllables. There are established DDK rate norms for each year of age through childhood and for adults with various underlying conditions. The patient's ability to repeat a word or syllable a number of times infers information about the lucidity and mobility of the tongue after glossectomy and reconstruction. Hsiao et al. used repetition rate as an objective evaluation of speech when comparing different methods of reconstruction after glossectomy and in a functional outcome analysis of glossectomy patients reconstructed with RFFF (Hsiao et al., 2002; Hsiao, Leu, & Lin, 2003). By relating repetition rate to the type of reconstruction used, they made observations about how the surgical rehabilitation method alters tongue movement and mobility.

A number of studies have used *ultrasound imaging* combined with perceptual evaluation to analyze the biomechanical nature of tongue movement during speech

(Bressmann et al., 2005; Rastadmehr, Bressmann, Smyth, & Irish, 2008). Rastadmehr et al. instructed patients to read the first four sentences of a passage with a variety of phonemes to mimic everyday conversational speech (Rastadmehr et al., 2008). Ultrasound imaging of the tongue was conducted during the passage recital, and information about tongue velocity and movement was recorded. Reading time as a quantitative perceptual measure was recorded and was related to tongue velocity and mobility (Rastadmehr et al., 2008). Other studies used clinical tongue mobility testing to relate speech deficits to lack of lucidity or mobility of the tongue (Matsui et al., 2007; Shin et al., 2012; Thankappan et al., 2011; Yun et al., 2010). Matsui et al. measured tongue mobility in relation to intelligibility and subjective speech evaluation (Matsui et al., 2007).

Acoustic evaluation includes the analysis of characteristics of vowel and diphthong sounds, i.e., duration, first and second formants and fundamental frequency, and sibilant sounds, i.e., spectral moments and frication duration, from speech samples (Laaksonen, 2010; Laaksonen, Rieger, Harris, & Seikaly, 2010). Acoustic characteristics correspond to the function of different tongue movements for diphthongs and position vowels, helping to determine the reasons for reduction in intelligibility of speech. Formants are the resonant harmonics in the speech spectrum and are described as being the characteristic partials of individual's speech (Atal & Hanaver, 1971). Formant frequencies objectively measure approximation between various portions of the oral cavity and the oropharynx. Although there are infinite numbers of formants, only the first three are of clinical use (de Carvalho-Teles, Sennes, & Gielow, 2008). First formant frequency (F1) is related to the vertical displacement of the tongue and F2 with the horizontal displacement of tongue, while F3 is related to the size of the oral and oropharyngeal cavity (de Carvalho-Teles et al., 2008). Information about the effects of size, site, and method of reconstruction on speech may be acquired by evaluating changes in these frequencies before and after resection and surgical rehabilitation and over time (Laaksonen, 2010; Laaksonen et al., 2010).

It has been shown that the larger the acoustic area, the greater the articulatory space, enabling a more precise articulation and a better intelligibility of speech (Laaksonen, 2010). Laaksonen et al. were able to define whether RFFF reconstruction of hemiglossectomy defects reduces the ability of patients to produce vowel sounds as indicated by vowel space area. The same group reported on the effect of resection and reconstruction with an RFFF on the acoustics of sibilants by measuring certain spectral and temporal characteristics. They were able to reflect on functional changes in the ability to articulate (Laaksonen et al., 2010). Sibilants require detailed somatosensory feedback (tactile and proprioceptive) and precise muscular movements, being some of the most challenging sounds to produce (Reichard et al., 2012). This in turn allows the evaluator to understand how different reconstruction methods alter tongue movement and ability to articulate.

Subjective assessment usually includes self-reported questionnaires about speech function. Subjective patient information evaluates speech outcome from the patient's perspective and allows the evaluator to measure the patient's satisfaction with final outcome. More importantly, subjective data infers information about the quality of speech and the patient's overall quality of life based on the speech deficits present.

Swallowing: Determinants of Functional Outcome

The tumor site, size, and extent of its excision, as well as the method of reconstruction, determine the adverse effects of surgery on swallowing (Hsiao et al., 2002; Logemann et al., 1993; Nicoletti, Soutar, Jackson, Wrench, & Robertson, 2004; O'Connell et al., 2008; Pauloski et al., 1993). In addition, the use of multimodal therapy including postoperative radiotherapy has been shown to affect swallowing outcomes (Shin et al., 2012; Thankappan et al., 2011). Studies on swallowing impairment are common and dependent on tumor site and size (Hara, Gellrich, Duker, Schön, Nilius, et al. 2003; Nicoletti, Soutar, Jackson, Wrench, & Robertson, 2004; Pauloski et al., 2004; Su, 2003; Thoné, Karengera, Siciliano, & Reychler, 2003). Borggreven et al. found a significant positive correlation between large tongue tumors or extensive resections and increased morbidity from dysphagia (Borggreven et al., 2007). Patients with smaller resections showed better swallowing outcomes, while patients with base of tongue resections showed worse outcomes with regard to tumor site (Nicoletti, Soutar, Jackson, Wrench, & Robertson, 2004). Furthermore, patients with resection of the oral tongue and floor of the mouth experienced problems in the oral phase, while patients after resection of the base of tongue encountered swallowing dysfunction in the pharyngeal phase (Hara et al., 2003; Nicoletti, Soutar, Jackson, Wrench, & Robertson, 2004; Pauloski et al., 2004). Hara et al. showed that regardless of the type of free flap used, the larger the resection, the greater was the impairment of the tongue movement due to scar formation. They also showed that patients who underwent the most anterior (lingual tip) had greater decreases in global tongue mobility than those who underwent lateral and posterior resections. Accordingly, resection of the anterior tongue and floor of the mouth had more impairment in swallowing than patients with resection of the lateral tongue or base of tongue (Hara et al., 2003).

Similar to speech outcome, the effect of the type of reconstruction on swallowing is not clear (Hsiao et al., 2002; Khariwala et al., 2007; Logemann et al., 1993; Nicoletti, Soutar, Jackson, Wrench, & Robertson, 2004; O'Connell et al., 2008; Pauloski et al., 1993; Su, 2003). Hsiao et al. reported better swallowing in patients with RFFF reconstruction in terms of larger bolus volume and better ingestion rate compared to those with primary closure following hemiglossectomy of oral tongue (Hsiao et al., 2002). The same group used videofluoroscopy (VFS) studies to compare swallowing function of patients after hemiglossectomy and reconstruction with primary closure or RFFF. They found nearly normal patterns of swallowing in patients reconstructed with RFFF. These patients were able to make good tongue-palate contact, facilitating the sealing of the posterior pharyngeal sphincter and preventing premature spilling of the bolus (Hsiao, Leu, Chang, & Lee, 2003). Sue et al. showed no significant difference in swallowing outcome between patients who underwent hemiglossectomy and reconstruction with RFFF or PMF (Su, 2003). Similarly, there was no significant difference in swallowing outcome between RFFF and ALTF reconstruction in patients after subtotal glossectomy of the oral tongue (de Vicente et al., 2008). Hence, the type of reconstruction that allows for better swallowing outcomes remains elusive. It is evident that further research is required to fully understand the method of reconstruction required to surgically treat specific tongue tumors based on size and site.

With regard to multimodal therapy, including the use of postoperative radiotherapy, significantly higher proportion of patients who had adjuvant treatments had restricted tongue mobility and diet (Thankappan et al., 2011). On subjective examination, Shin et al. found that postoperative radiotherapy was related to poorer swallowing function after partial glossectomy and RFFF (Shin et al., 2012). In addition, radiotherapy may induce late complications such as subcutaneous fibrosis, mucosal edema, trismus, and salivary gland atrophy (Bokhari & Wang, 2007; Kazi et al., 2008; Pauloski et al., 1994).

Swallowing: Assessment Methods

Various methods are used to evaluate swallowing function and impairment, including objective radiological and clinical assesments, as well as, targeted patient questionnaires on swallowing deficits. Objective evaluations include the use of videofluoroscopic and modified barium swallowing (VFS/MBS) studies (Brown, 2010; O'Connell et al., 2008; Rieger, 2007; Seikaly, 2008; Uwiera et al., 2004). VFS studies are currently the preferred objective assessment methods in most institutions because it permits the visualization of bolus flow in relation to structural movement throughout the upper aerodigestive tract in real-time (Argon et al., 2004; Pauloski et al., 1994; Shaw et al., 2004). Further, clinicians are able to observe the effects of various bolus volumes, bolus textures, and compensatory strategies on swallowing physiology. Hence, VFS studies help to determine how tumor site and method of reconstruction affect tongue movement and swallowing (Hsiao, Leu, Chang, & Lee, 2003).

A number of studies used a variety of quantitative swallowing and tongue mobility measures to evaluate VFS studies (Brown, 2010; O'Connell et al., 2008; Rieger et al., 2006; Uwiera et al., 2004). Brown et al. reported on swallowing impairment in patients with resection of the anterior two-thirds of the tongue and reconstruction with RFFF (Brown, 2010). They were able to make standardized conclusions on how RFFF reconstruction of anterior tongue resections affected the oral and pharyngeal phase of swallowing. In addition, this study evaluated swallowing function postoperatively for 12 months and used VFS studies to show changes in swallowing impairment (Brown, 2010).

Clinical evaluations rely on functional tests or grading systems to rate the method, time required, and type of food intake (de Vicente et al., 2008; Hsiao et al., 2002; Hsiao, Leu, & Lin, 2003; Su, 2003; Thankappan et al., 2011; Yun et al., 2010). Hsiao et al. used functional tests that enabled them to determine the swallowing outcomes of patients with hemiglossectomy defects reconstructed with RFFF, in addition to comparing the swallowing outcomes between primary closure and RFFF reconstruction (Hsiao et al., 2002; Hsiao, Leu, & Lin, 2003). The same group used information on dietary habits relative to the results of the functional tests to further understand how RFFF reconstruction affected swallow outcomes (Hsiao, Leu, & Lin, 2003). When comparing lateral arm free flap (LAFF) reconstruction to RFFF of tongue defects, Thankappan et al. based swallowing functional outcome on dietary characteristics: unrestricted, soft, and liquid. Patients with less diet restrictions and more regular diet had better swallowing outcomes (Thankappan et al., 2011). A number of studies (de Vicente et al., 2008; Su, 2003) used a 1–7 scale to evaluate swallowing objectively as previously described by Teichgraeber in 1985 (Teichgraeber, Bowman, & Goepfert, 1985). Su et al. clinically evaluated swallowing outcomes of patients with reconstruction with either RFFF or PMF where the average swallow rating was related to the extent of resection and the type of flap used to reconstruct glossectomy defects (Su, 2003). Similarly, RFFF and ALTF reconstructions of hemiglossectomy defects were compared to objectively identify changes in functional outcomes of swallowing (de Vicente et al., 2008).

Subjective assessment by means of questionnaires has been used to determine swallow outcomes. Su et al. used a questionnaire on the consistency of the diet to analyze the effect of the flap type used on the swallowing outcomes. Liquid consistency diets were related to lower swallowing outcomes and patients with larger resections, such as in patients with total glossectomy, while patients with hemiglossectomy had better swallowing outcomes and were able to eat semisolid or regular diets (Su, 2003). Kazi et al. used the M.D. Anderson Dysphagia Inventory (MDADI) which is a validated questionnaire designed to assess swallowing dysfunction based on global, emotional, functional, and physical scores (Kazi et al., 2008). Similarly Shin et al. used the MDADI as a subjective means of evaluating swallow outcomes after hemiglossectomy and reconstruction with RFFF (Shin et al., 2012). Patient-reported scales or questionnaires are helpful in assessing how patients view the outcome of their swallowing as a result of treatment and how changes in swallowing affected their quality of life (Kazi et al., 2008).

Evidence for Primary Closure

When considering the method of reconstruction of glossectomy defects, the main goal is to optimize speech and swallow outcomes. There is evidence in the literature that surgical resection of less than half of the tongue typically results in minimal and temporary dysfunction in speech and swallow (Michiwaki et al., 1992; Pauloski et al., 1998). Furthermore, there is evidence to support that small defects remaining after ablative surgery may be closed primarily without significant functional deficiency (Bressmann et al., 2005;Chuanjun, 2002 ; Hsiao et al., 2002 ; McConnel et al., 1998). This no doubt will affect the patient's everyday quality of life. McConnel et al. reported on a multi-institutional prospective study evaluating speech and swallow outcomes after oral and base of tongue glossectomy, based on the method of reconstruction: primary closure, distal myocutaneous flaps, and microvascular free flaps (McConnel et al., 1998). This evaluation included VFS studies for swallow function, speech intelligibility, and sentence articulation testing. Patients who had primary closure were more efficient at swallowing liquids and had less pharyngeal residue, a longer oral transit time with paste, and higher conversational intelligibility than patients who underwent reconstruction with a distal flap. Compared with patients who underwent reconstruction with a free flap, those who had primary closure had more efficient swallowing of liquids, less pharyngeal residue, and shorter pharyngeal delay times with paste (McConnel et al., 1998). These results indicate that the bulk of a muscle skin flap may be considered as a factor interfering with function in oral cavity and oropharyngeal reconstruction. They showed that a flap could be acting as an adynamic segment that impairs the driving force of the remaining tongue, thereby reducing the swallowing efficiency. This flap may also reduce the fine control of the tongue for speech (McConnel et al., 1998). They concluded that with relatively small resections of the oral tongue (30%) and tongue base (60%), there is no significant improvement in speech and swallowing efficiency between patients having flaps and patients with primary closure (McConnel et al., 1998).

Chuanjun et al. evaluated articulation intelligibility in patients with minor glossectomy or hemiglossectomy of T1 and T2 tongue cancer tumors reconstructed with either primary closure or vascularized flaps (Chuanjun, 2002). The articulation intelligibility was better in patients who were not receiving grafts compared to those with grafts. For patients who underwent primary closure, the intelligibility of articulation was significantly higher in blade portion, mid portion, and rear portion glossal sounds (Chuanjun, 2002). These results imply that the scar formation of the reconstructive flaps reduced the flexibility and mobility of the residual and, in turn, intensified articulatory impairment in patients who underwent reconstructive surgery. In addition, the remaining hemitongue reconstructed using RFFF without innervated muscle cannot produce voluntary movements. However, hemiglossectomy without reconstruction leaves a half-intact tongue, which may be more flexible in speaking movements than a reconstructed tongue. The residual hemitongue can compensate for the missing tongue to a great extent, as the articulation intelligibility scores indicate. The reconstruction with flaps, which interferes with the flexibility and mobility of the tongue, contributed to articulatory impairment. Therefore, if speech is the outcome of interest, reconstruction may be unnecessary for hemiglossectomy or partial glossectomy within the hemitongue (Chuanjun, 2002).

Hsiao et al. compared the postoperative speech and swallowing functions of patients who underwent RFFF reconstruction or primary closure after hemiglossectomy of T1–T3 tumors of the tongue (Hsiao et al., 2002). Speech quality, including intelligibility and articulation, was better in patients with primary closure. However, the bolus volume and ingestion rate in deglutition were better in those with flap reconstruction. Patients who underwent primary closure of the defect retained a small but freely movable tongue. The excellent mobility allowed for good speech, but the tongue displacement and volume loss resulted in less effective transport of food into the hypopharynx. This indicates that the volume and mobility of the reconstructed tongue determine the functional results of deglutition and speech in a hemiglossectomized patient. The flap increases bulk, thus improving pharyngeal clearance by maintaining the tongue-to-mouth roof contact that is necessary in the swallowing process, however hinders articulation by restricting the mobility of the remaining portion of the normal tongue (Hsiao et al., 2002).

For partial glossectomy defects without involvement of the tip, floor of the mouth, or base of tongue, free flap reconstruction does not appear to improve post-operative function over primary closure (Chuanjun, 2002). Three-dimensional echography shows a certain degree of lingual asymmetry, as a result of primary closure, can be compensated for quite successfully (Bressmann et al., 2007). The adynamic nature of the free flap may interfere with mobility and symmetry of the remaining tongue, thus accentuating the speech impairment (Bressmann et al., 2007). While the decision to use flap reconstruction in a case is obviously at the surgeon's discretion based on the extent of resection and the nature of the defect to be repaired, it is important to consider the use of primary closure where possible, especially if it is likely to improve functional outcomes (Chuanjun, 2002; McConnel et al., 1998; Zuydam et al., 2005).

Evidence for Free Flap Reconstruction

Microvascular free flap reconstruction represents a major advance in head and neck surgery (Hidalgo & Pusic, 2002; Urken, 2003). To date, the reliability of microvascular head and neck reconstruction is well established, and some authors have reported free flap success percentages over 95%, following careful patient selection (Dassonville et al., 2008; Urken, 2003). Because of better outcome in terms of function, cosmesis, and consequently a better quality of life, many have advocated the use of free vascularized flaps, such as RFFF, to reconstruct soft tissue defects in the oral cavity and oropharynx (Borggreven et al., 2007; Bozec et al., 2007; Chien, Su, Hwang, & Chuang, 2006; Hara et al., 2003; Khariwala et al., 2007; Seikaly et al., 2003). Surgical resection of less than half of the tongue typically results in minimal and only temporary deficits in speech and swallowing. Small defects after ablative surgery usually close primarily without significant functional deficiency (Chuanjun, 2002; Hsiao et al., 2002; McConnel et al., 1998). However, larger surgical defects leave patients with significant functional morbidity (Yu & Robb, 2005). Therefore, it is evident that flap reconstruction usually is required if more than half of the tongue is resected (Hsiao, Leu, Chang, & Lee, 2003).

In patients who undergo hemiglossectomy and reconstruction with free flap transfer, the remaining oropharyngeal tissue is relatively large, and the majority of patients recover speech and eating functions, and this allows them to live a normal life. Hsiao et al. studied the swallowing function of patients with T2–T3 tumors in the anterior two-thirds of the lateral tongue and who underwent hemiglossectomy with either primary closure of the defect or RFFF reconstruction (Hsiao, Leu, Chang, & Lee, 2003). With flap reconstruction, patients easily could lift the tongue and make good contact with the entire palate. They were able to seal the posterior pharyngeal sphincter by elevation of the reconstructed tongue, approximating it to the soft palate, so that premature spilling of the bolus rarely happened. Their swallowing pattern was nearly normal. They suggested that although the reconstructed flap is nonfunctional, it provides bulk and helps the remaining tongue to complete the swallow. The authors concluded that it is better to reconstruct with a RFFF when more than half of the tongue is resected to restore tongue volume and swallowing efficiency (Hsiao, Leu, Chang, & Lee, 2003). Similarly, other studies have shown that primary closure of partial or hemiglossectomy defects provides better tongue mobility to allow for better speech (Bressmann et al., 2007; Chuanjun, 2002; Hsiao et al., 2002; McConnel et al., 1998). It is evident that swallowing outcomes are better when more volume is added to the remaining small mobile tongue (Hsiao, Leu, Chang, & Lee, 2003).

The same group evaluated speech and swallow outcomes of patients after hemiglossectomy of the anteriolateral tongue and reconstruction with RFFF (Hsiao, Leu, & Lin, 2003). The majority of patients scored between 3 (difficult to understand) and 5 (intelligible speech with noticeable errors), with 50% of patients scoring 5 and over half of the patients had distorted articulation which was acceptable or improved with multiple repetitions (Hsiao, Leu, & Lin, 2003). In addition, swallowing function among these patients did not differ significantly from that of controls based on measures of bolus volume, duration of deglutition, and ingestion rate (Hsiao, Leu, & Lin, 2003). The RFFF reconstruction technique they used provided bulk necessary for good deglutition, although improvements would be required to further enhance speech (Hsiao, Leu, & Lin, 2003). Thankappan et al. reported on the functional outcomes of patients who underwent partial glossectomy for T1–T3 tumors of the lateral border of the tongue and reconstruction with LAFF (Thankappan et al., 2011). In their study, speech was normal or nearly normal in all patients, and tongue movement was not grossly restricted in the majority of patients. Furthermore, most of the patients were able to consume an unrestricted diet, while a minority were restricted to soft foods (Thankappan et al., 2011). They concluded that LAFF is an excellent flap option for the reconstruction of partial glossectomy defects without involvement of the floor of the mouth (Thankappan et al., 2011).

Uwiera et al. prospectively evaluated the functional outcomes of patients who underwent hemiglossectomy of T2–T3 of tongue tumors and RFFF reconstruction (Uwiera et al., 2004). Their patients were evaluated preoperatively and postoperatively, at 1 and 6 months after surgery. There was no significant difference across any of the evaluation times for sentence intelligibility (Uwiera et al., 2004). With respect to swallowing, analysis revealed fewer instances of laryngeal penetration with liquids postoperatively, no incidence of penetration for either pudding or cookie bolus, and no incidence of aspiration at any of the evaluation times (Uwiera et al., 2004). In addition, there were no significant differences in any of the oral preparatory swallowing parameters (bolus hold, bolus form, mastication, lip closure) or the oral phase swallowing parameters (bolus control, prolonged transit time, oral stasis) across treatment times. They concluded that RFFF provides functional speech which can consistently achieve preoperative levels and the necessary structure to restore the ability of the patient to consume a fairly *normal diet* (Uwiera et al., 2004). Similarly, Brown et al. showed that there was significant decline in swallowing of liquid at 1 month after hemiglossectomy of the anterior two-thirds of the tongue and RFFF reconstruction. This was shown to be due to premature laryngeal penetrations and a higher number of swallowing attempts to clear the bolus; however, all VFS parameters returned to preoperative levels after 1 year (Brown, 2010).

Although there is decline in speech and swallowing outcomes in the postoperative phase, patients with flap reconstruction of partial or hemiglossectomy defects recover and reach preoperative outcomes with time (Brown, 2010; Uwiera et al., 2004). The use of free flaps is a reliable and efficient method of reconstruction, especially when tongue bulk is required (Brown, 2010; Hsiao, Leu, Chang, & Lee, 2003; Hsiao, Leu, & Lin, 2003; Seikaly, 2008; Uwiera et al., 2004). However, the use of free flaps has been most highlighted for larger defects which are not amendable to primary closure (Seikaly, 2008; Urken et al., 1994; Yu & Robb, 2005). For partial and hemiglossectomy defects after resection of T1–T2 tumors, further evidence is required to establish functional outcome benefits of free flaps as compared to primary closure, specifically, with regard to speech and swallow outcomes, as well as overall morbidity caused by the use of free flaps.

Functional Reconstruction

Successful tongue reconstruction involves more than satisfactory wound healing and flap survival (Urken et al., 1994). Mobility and volume of the oral tongue are essential for speech and swallowing (Urken et al., 1994). Hence, the goal of functional reconstruction after partial or hemiglossectomy is to maximize mobility of the residual tongue and to maintain its shape and volume within the oral cavity by primary closure or by introducing free flaps (Brown, 2010; de Vicente et al., 2008;Urken et al., 1994 ; Urken & Biller, 1994 ; Uwiera et al., 2004).

The quality of speech after hemiglossectomy is more a function of tongue mobility than volume (Hsiao et al., 2002). It has been noted that preservation of the tip of the tongue and the floor of the mouth, excision of cancer located laterally, and smaller excision have better speech outcomes (Matsui et al., 2007; Sun et al., 2007). This can be ascribed to greater mobility of the residual tongue and a greater ability to articulate (Matsui et al., 2007). Furthermore, as compared to RFFF reconstruction, patients after primary closure of hemiglossectomy defects show better speech outcomes (Chuanjun, 2002; Hsiao et al., 2002). This has been attributed to the fact that the freely movable residual tongue maintains good mobility and allows for better speech (Bressmann et al., 2007; Chuanjun, 2002; Hsiao et al., 2002). Hence, primary closure of partial or hemiglossectomy defects remains a very simple yet effective technique to optimize speech outcomes by maintaining greater mobility of the residual tongue.

Anterior resection including floor of the mouth significantly reduces the mobility of the whole tongue and limits tip elevation to touch the alveolar ridge or palate, in turn, intensifying the speech and swallow dysfunction (Matsui et al., 2007; Rieger,

2007; Sun et al., 2007). The use of a bilobed design of RFFF to separately reconstruct the oral tongue and the floor of the mouth has also been advocated to improve the functional outcomes (Urken et al., 1994; Urken & Biller, 1994; Uwiera et al., 2004). Speech outcomes in patients with partial or hemiglossectomy defects reconstructed with RFFF regain preoperative levels after 1 year and remain acceptable (Brown, 2010; Uwiera et al., 2004). In addition, as compared to patients who had primary closure, patients who had RFFF reconstruction of hemiglossectomy defects had a tongue-palate contact that is required to complete a swallow and showed nearly normal swallowing pattern (Hsiao, Leu, Chang, & Lee, 2003; Hsiao, Leu, & Lin, 2003). Although the flap is nonfunctional, it adds the required bulk for the residual tongue to complete an efficient swallow (Brown, 2010; Hsiao, Leu, Chang, & Lee, 2003). Hence, the use of a thin and pliable free flap, such as RFFF, ALTF, and LAFF, can facilitate good recovery of intelligibility, articulation, and swallowing by providing volume required to fill the oral cavity (Matsui et al., 2009; Sun et al., 2007; Thankappan et al., 2011; Uwiera et al., 2004).

The complexity of the tongue structure limits the possibilities for functional reconstruction (Engel, 2010). In fact, the ideal method for reconstruction of partial or hemiglossectomy defects remains elusive. Functional reconstruction is aimed at optimizing speech and swallow outcomes. There is evidence for both primary closure and free flap reconstruction in the treatment of partial or hemiglossectomy defects, based on the mobility and volume of the reconstructed residual tongue (de Vicente et al., 2008; Hsiao et al., 2002; Hsiao, Leu, Chang, & Lee, 2003; Hsiao, Leu, & Lin, 2003; Seikaly, 2008; Uwiera et al., 2004). When deciding for the best method of reconstruction, it is important to consider other factors. Older patients and patients with associated comorbid conditions are known to have poor functions as compared to their younger counterparts who have better healing and regeneration potential (Matsui et al., 2007; Nicoletti, Soutar, Jackson, Wrench, & Robertson, 2004). In addition, donor-site morbidity associated with the use of free flaps presents a significant disadvantage to this method of reconstruction (de Vicente et al., 2008; Huang, Chen, Huang, Mardini, & Feng, 2004). When taken together, primary closure presents an ideal treatment due to its technical simplicity and lack of donor-site morbidity. However, free flap reconstruction is often better in providing overall swallow outcomes (Hara et al., 2003; Uwiera et al., 2004). For this reason both primary closure and free flap reconstruction should be considered and employed for the surgical rehabilitation of partial and hemiglossectomy defects.

Conclusions

Patients who have tongue cancer and have experienced the effects of complicated treatment methods such as that which has been described above may suffer from problems of communication, nutrition, work-related difficulties, and maintaining relationships at home and with friends, along with issues of isolation, loneliness, possible depression, and fear of recurrence. However, overall functional speech and swallowing outcomes of partial or hemiglossectomy and reconstruction are influenced by multiple factors including tumor size, site, method of reconstruction, and the use of postoperative radiotherapy. Although there is significant decline in speech and swallow measures postoperatively, the majority of patients recover to preoperative levels. Speech and swallow outcomes are directly associated with the volume and degree of mobility remaining after surgical interventions. Surgical rehabilitation whether by primary closure or free flaps for the immediate reconstruction of the tongue after tumor resection should aim at the maintenance of the mobility of the residual tongue and restoration of tongue bulk, in order to optimize the recovery of speech and swallowing functions. Primary closure of partial and hemiglossectomy defects is beneficial in maintaining higher mobility of the residual tongue to optimize speech. On the other hand, free flap reconstruction allows for volume and bulk modifications to the residual tongue required to optimize swallowing. Hence, when contemplating the method of reconstruction, both primary closure and free flap reconstruction of partial or hemiglossectomy defects should be considered.

Presently, the literature shows a wide variation in the level of evidence, methodological design, and reporting of results. There is a lack of standardized classification of tongue defects and functional evaluation methods. Moreover, there is little evidence comparing the functional outcomes of patients with partial and hemiglossectomy defects reconstructed with primary closure or free flaps. For patients who present with T1–T2 tumors, further evidence is required to determine the best method of reconstruction that takes into account speech, swallowing, and overall patient quality of life and morbidity, including donor-site morbidity. Future research in this field should employ standardized and reliable evaluation methods of speech and swallowing outcomes to further explore these factors by using multiple modalities in well-designed cohort and longitudinal studies. In addition, future investigations should further examine the psychological effects of the various surgical treatments and interventions on the quality of life among tongue cancer patients by conducting a qualitative inquiry using a large sample of patients. Nevertheless, oncology professionals and dental clinicians and researchers working with these patients should gain valuable information and insight from the review that was presented in this chapter. Further understanding of these issues will ultimately reflect on quality of care and more comprehensive services to this population of cancer survivors.

References

Argon, M., Secil, Y., Duygun, U., Aydogdu, I., Kocacelebi, K., Ozkilic, H., & Ertekin, C. (2004). The value of scintigraphy in the evaluation of oropharyngeal dysphagia. *European Journal of Nuclear Medicine and Molecular Imaging*, *31*(1), 94–98. https://doi.org/10.1007/s00259-003-1276-0

Atal, B. S., & Hanaver, S. L. (1971). Speech analysis and synthesis by linear prediction of the speech wave. *The Journal of the Acoustical Society of America*, *50*(2), 637–655.

Bokhari, W. A., & Wang, S. J. (2007). Tongue reconstruction: Recent advances. *Current Opinion in Otolaryngology & Head and Neck Surgery, 15*(4), 202–207. https://doi.org/10.1097/MOO.0b013e3281fbd406

Borggreven, P. A., Verdonck-de Leeuw, I., Langendijk, J. A., Doornaert, P., Koster, M. N., de Bree, R., & Leemans, C. R. (2005). Speech outcome after surgical treatment for oral and oropharyngeal cancer: a longitudinal assessment of patients reconstructed by a microvascular flap. *Head & neck, 27*(9), 785–793.

Borggreven, P. A., Leeuw, I. V. D., Rinkel, R. N., Langendijk, J. A., Roos, J. C., David, E. F., ... & Leemans, C. R. (2007). Swallowing after major surgery of the oral cavity or oropharynx: a prospective and longitudinal assessment of patients treated by microvascular soft tissue reconstruction. *Head & neck, 29*(7), 638–647.

Bozec, A., Poissonnet, G., Converset, S., Lattes, L., Chamorey, E., Vallicionni, J., … Dassonville, O. (2007). Oropharyngeal reconstruction with radial forearm free flap: Functional results. *Revue De Laryngologie – Otologie – Rhinologie, 128*(1–2), 19–26.

Bressmann, T., Ackloo, E., Heng, C.-L., & Irish, J. C. (2007). Quantitative three-dimensional ultrasound imaging of partially resected tongues. *Head & Neck Surgery, 136*, 799–805.

Bressmann, T., Sader, R., Whitehill, T. L., & Samman, N. (2004). Consonant intelligibility and tongue motility in patients with partial glossectomy. *Journal of Oral and Maxillofacial Surgery, 62*(3), 298–303. https://doi.org/10.1016/j.joms.2003.04.017

Bressmann, T., Thind, P., Uy, C., Bollig, C., Gilbert, R. W., & Irish, J. C. (2005). Quantitative three-dimensional ultrasound analysis of tongue protrusion, grooving and symmetry: Data from 12 normal speakers and a partial glossectomy. *Clinical Linguistics & Phonetics, 19*(6–7), 573–588. https://doi.org/10.1080/02699200500113947

Brown, L. (2010). A longitudinal study of functional outcomes after surgical resection and microvascular reconstruction for oral cancer: Tongue mobility and swallowing function. *Yjoms, 68*(11), 2690–2700. https://doi.org/10.1016/j.joms.2010.05.004

Carvalho, A. L., Nishimoto, I. N., Califano, J. A., & Kowalski, L. P. (2004). Trends in incidence and prognosis for head and neck cancer in the United States: A site-specific analysis of the SEER database. *International Journal of Cancer, 114*(5), 806–816. https://doi.org/10.1002/ijc.20740

Chien, C. Y., Su, C. Y., Hwang, C. F., & Chuang, H. C. (2006). Ablation of advanced tongue or base of tongue cancer and reconstruction with free flap: Functional outcomes. *European Journal of Surgical Oncology, 32*, 353–357.

Chong, V. (2005). Oral cavity cancer. *Cancer Imaging : the Official Publication of the International Cancer Imaging Society, 5 Spec No A*, S49–52. https://doi.org/10.1102/1470-7330.2005.0029

Chuanjun, C. (2002). Speech after partial glossectomy: A comparison between reconstruction and nonreconstruction patients. *Journal of Oral and Maxillofacial Surgery, 60*(4), 404–407. https://doi.org/10.1053/joms.2002.31228

Colangelo, L. A., Logemann, J. A., & Rademaker, A. W. (2000). Tumor size and pretreatment speech and swallowing in patients with resectable tumors. *Otolaryngology–Head and Neck Surgery : Official Journal of American Academy of Otolaryngology-Head and Neck Surgery, 122*(5), 653–661.

Costa Bandeira, A. K., Azevedo, E. H., Vartanian, J. G., Nishimoto, I. N., Kowalski, L. P., & Carrara-de Angelis, E. (2008). Quality of life related to swallowing after tongue cancer treatment. *Dysphagia, 23*(2), 183–192. Epub 2007 Nov 13. PMID: 17999111. https://doi.org/10.1007/s00455-007-9124-1

Dassonville, O., Poissonnet, G., Chamorey, E., Vallicioni, J., Demard, F., Santini, J., … Bozec, A. (2008). Head and neck reconstruction with free flaps: A report on 213 cases. *European Archives of Oto-Rhino-Laryngology, 265*(1), 85–95. https://doi.org/10.1007/s00405-007-0410-1

de Carvalho-Teles, V., Sennes, L. U., & Gielow, I. (2008). Speech evaluation after palatal augmentation in patients undergoing glossectomy. *Archives of Otolaryngology–Head & Neck Surgery, 134*(10), 1066–1070. https://doi.org/10.1001/archotol.134.10.1066

de Vicente, J. C., de Villalaín, L., Torre, A., & Peña, I. (2008). Microvascular free tissue transfer for tongue reconstruction after hemiglossectomy: A functional assessment of radial forearm versus anterolateral thigh flap. *Journal of Oral and Maxillofacial Surgery : Official Journal of the American Association of Oral and Maxillofacial Surgeons, 66*(11), 2270–2275. https://doi.org/10.1016/j.joms.2008.01.018

Dodds, W. J., Logemann, J. A., & Stewart, E. T. (1990). Radiologic assessment of abnormal oral and pharyngeal phases of swallowing. *AJR. American Journal of Roentgenology, 154*(5), 965–974. https://doi.org/10.2214/ajr.154.5.2108570

Dwivedi, R. C., Kazi, R. A., Agrawal, N., & Nutting, C. M. (2009). Evaluation of speech outcomes following treatment of oral and oropharyngeal cancers. *Cancer Treatment Reviews, 35*(5), 417–424.

Engel, H. (2010). A strategic approach for tongue reconstruction to achieve predictable and improved functional and aesthetic outcomes. *Plastic and Reconstructive Surgery, 126*(6), 1967–1977. https://doi.org/10.1097/PRS.0b013e3181f44742

Gadesmann, M., & Miller, N. (2008). Reliability of speech diadochokinetic test measurement. *International Journal of Language & Communication Disorders, 43*(1), 41–54. https://doi.org/10.1080/13682820701234444

Hamlet, S. L., Mathog, R. H., Patterson, R. L., & Fleming, S. M. (1990). Tongue mobility in speech after partial glossectomy. *Head & Neck, 12*(3), 210–217. https://doi.org/10.1002/hed.2880120304

Hara, I., Gellrich, N. C., Duker, J., Schön, R., Fakler, O., Smelzeisen, R., … Satoru, O. (2003). Swallowing and speech function after intraoral soft tissue reconstruction with lateral upper arm free flap and radial forearm free flap. *British Journal of Oral & Maxillofacial Surgery, 41*(3), 161–169. https://doi.org/10.1016/S0266-4356(03)00068-8

Hara, I., Gellrich, N. C., Duker, J., Schön, R., Nilius, M., Fakler, O., … Honda, T. (2003). Evaluation of swallowing function after intraoral soft tissue reconstruction with microvascular free flaps. *International Journal of Oral and Maxillofacial Surgery, 32*(6), 593–599. https://doi.org/10.1054/ijom.2002.0436

Hartl, D. M., Dauchy, S., Escande, C., Bretagne, E., Janot, F., & Kolb, F. (2009). Quality of life after free-flap tongue reconstruction. *The Journal of Laryngology & Otology, 123*(05), 550–554. https://doi.org/10.1017/S0022215108003629

Hidalgo, D. A., & Pusic, A. L. (2002). Free-flap mandibular reconstruction: A 10-year follow-up study. *Plastic and Reconstructive Surgery, 110*(2), 438–449. discussion 450–1.

Hsiao, H.-T., Leu, Y.-S., Chang, S.-H., & Lee, J.-T. (2003). Swallowing function in patients who underwent hemiglossectomy: Comparison of primary closure and free radial forearm flap reconstruction with videofluoroscopy. *Annals of Plastic Surgery, 50*(5), 450–455. https://doi.org/10.1097/01.SAP.0000044147.09310.E8

Hsiao, H.-T., Leu, Y.-S., & Lin, C.-C. (2002). Primary closure versus radial forearm flap reconstruction after hemiglossectomy: Functional assessment of swallowing and speech. *Annals of Plastic Surgery, 49*(6), 612–616. https://doi.org/10.1097/01.SAP.0000024760.06545.E7

Hsiao, H.-T., Leu, Y.-S., & Lin, C.-C. (2003). Tongue reconstruction with free radial forearm flap after hemiglossectomy: A functional assessment. *Journal of Reconstructive Microsurgery, 19*(3), 137–142. https://doi.org/10.1055/s-2003-39824

Huang, C.-H., Chen, H.-C., Huang, Y.-L., Mardini, S., & Feng, G.-M. (2004). Comparison of the radial forearm flap and the thinned anterolateral thigh cutaneous flap for reconstruction of tongue defects: An evaluation of donor-site morbidity. *Plastic and Reconstructive Surgery, 114*(7), 1704–1710. https://doi.org/10.1097/01.PRS.0000142476.36975.07

Kazi, R., Prasad, V., Venkitaraman, R., Nutting, C. M., Clarke, P., Rhys-Evans, P., & Harrington, K. J. (2008). Questionnaire analysis of swallowing-related outcomes following glossectomy. *ORL; Journal for Oto-Rhino-Laryngology and Its Related Specialties, 70*(3), 151–155. https://doi.org/10.1159/000124287

Khariwala, S. S., Vivek, P. P., Lorenz, R. R., Esclamado, R. M., Wood, B., Strome, M., & Alam, D. S. (2007). Swallowing outcomes after microvascular head and neck reconstruction: A prospective review of 191 cases. *The Laryngoscope, 117*(8), 1359–1363. https://doi.org/10.1097/MLG.0b013e3180621109

Laaksonen, J.-P. (2010). Speech after radial forearm free flap reconstruction of the tongue: A longitudinal acoustic study of vowel and diphthong sounds. *Clinical Linguistics & Phonetics, 24*(1), 41–54. https://doi.org/10.3109/02699200903340758

Laaksonen, J.-P., Rieger, J., Harris, J., & Seikaly, H. (2010). A longitudinal acoustic study of the effects of the radial forearm free flap reconstruction on sibilants produced by tongue cancer patients. *Clinical Linguistics & Phonetics, 25*(4), 253–264. https://doi.org/10.3109/02699206.2010.525681

List, M. A., Stracks, J., Colangelo, L., Butler, P., Ganzenko, N., Lundy, D., … Vokes, E. E. (2000). How do head and neck cancer patients prioritize treatment outcomes before initiating treatment? *Journal of Clinical Oncology, 18*(4), 877–884.

Loewen, I. J., Boliek, C. A., Harris, J., & Seikaly, H. (2010). Oral sensation and function: A comparison of patients with innervated radial forearm free flap reconstruction to healthy matched controls. *Head & Neck, 32*, 85–95. Loewen – 2009 – Wiley Online Library.

Logemann, J. A., Pauloski, B. R., Rademaker, A. W., McConnel, F. M., Heiser, M. A., Cardinale, S., … Johnson, J. (1993). Speech and swallow function after tonsil/base of tongue resection with primary closure. *Journal of Speech and Hearing Research, 36*(5), 918–926.

Matsui, Y., Ohno, K., Yamashita, Y., & Takahashi, K. (2007). Factors influencing postoperative speech function of tongue cancer patients following reconstruction with fasciocutaneous/myocutaneous flaps—A multicenter study. *International Journal of Oral and Maxillofacial Surgery, 36*(7), 601–609. https://doi.org/10.1016/j.ijom.2007.01.014

Matsui, Y., Shirota, T., Yamashita, Y., & Ohno, K. (2009). Analyses of speech intelligibility in patients after glossectomy and reconstruction with fasciocutaneous/myocutaneous flaps. *International Journal of Oral and Maxillofacial Surgery, 38*(4), 339–345.

McConnel, F. M., Pauloski, B. R., Logemann, J. A., Rademaker, A. W., Colangelo, L., Shedd, D., … Johnson, J. (1998). Functional results of primary closure vs flaps in oropharyngeal reconstruction: A prospective study of speech and swallowing. *Archives of Otolaryngology–Head & Neck Surgery, 124*(6), 625–630.

Michi, K. (2003). Functional evaluation of cancer surgery in oral and maxillofacial region: Speech function. *International Journal of Clinical Oncology, 8*(1), 1–17. https://doi.org/10.1007/s101470300000

Michiwaki, Y., Schmelzeisen, R., Hacki, T., & Michi, K. (1992). Articulatory function in glossectomized patients with immediate reconstruction using a free jejunum flap. *Journal of Cranio-Maxillo-Facial Surgery : Official Publication of the European Association for Cranio-Maxillo-Facial Surgery, 20*(5), 203–210.

Nicoletti, G., Soutar, D. S., Jackson, M. S., Wrench, A. A., & Robertson, G. (2004). Chewing and swallowing after surgical treatment for oral cancer: Functional evaluation in 196 selected cases. *Plastic and Reconstructive Surgery, 114*(2), 329–338.

Nicoletti, G., Soutar, D. S., Jackson, M. S., Wrench, A. A., Robertson, G., & Robertson, C. (2004). Objective assessment of speech after surgical treatment for oral cancer: Experience from 196 selected cases. *Plastic and Reconstructive Surgery, 113*(1), 114–125. https://doi.org/10.1097/01.PRS.0000095937.45812.84

O'Connell, D. A., Rieger, J., Harris, J. R., Dziegielewski, P., Zalmanowitz, J., Sytsanko, A., … Seikaly, H. (2008). Swallowing function in patients with base of tongue cancers treated with primary surgery and reconstructed with a modified radial forearm free flap. *Archives of Otolaryngology--Head & Neck Surgery, 134*(8), 857–864. https://doi.org/10.1001/archotol.134.8.857

Pauloski, B. R., Logemann, J. A., Colangelo, L. A., Rademaker, A. W., McConnel, F. M. S., Heiser, M. A., … Esclamado, R. (1998). Surgical variables affecting speech in treated patients with oral and oropharyngeal cancer. *The Laryngoscope, 108*(6), 908–916. https://doi.org/10.1097/00005537-199806000-00022

Pauloski, B. R., Logemann, J. A., & Rademaker, A. W. (1994). Speech and swallowing function after oral and oropharyngeal resections: One-year follow-up. *Head & Neck, 16*(4), 313–322. Pauloski – 2006 – Wiley Online Library.

Pauloski, B. R., Logemann, J. A., Rademaker, A. W., McConnel, F. M., Heiser, M. A., Cardinale, S., … Baker, T. (1993). Speech and swallowing function after anterior tongue and floor of

mouth resection with distal flap reconstruction. *Journal of Speech and Hearing Research, 36*(2), 267–276.
Pauloski, B. R., Rademaker, A. W., Logemann, J. A., McConnel, F. M. S., Heiser, M. A., Cardinale, S., … Beery, Q. (2004). Surgical variables affecting swallowing in patients treated for oral/oropharyngeal cancer. *Head & Neck, 26*(7), 625–636. https://doi.org/10.1002/hed.20013
Radford, K., Woods, H., & Lowe, D. (2004). A UK multi-centre pilot study of speech and swallowing outcomes following head and neck cancer. *Clinical Otolaryngology & Allied Sciences, 29*(4), 376–381. Radford – 2004 – Wiley Online Library.
Rastadmehr, O., Bressmann, T., Smyth, R., & Irish, J. C. (2008). Increased midsagittal tongue velocity as indication of articulatory compensation in patients with lateral partial glossectomies. *Head & Neck, 30*(6), 718–726. https://doi.org/10.1002/hed.20772
Reichard, R., Stone, M., & Woo, J. (2012). Motion of apical and laminal/s/in normal and post-glossectomy speakers. *Journal of the Acoustical Society of America, 131*, 3346–3350.
Rieger, J. M. (2007). Functional outcomes after surgical reconstruction of the base of tongue using the radial forearm free flap in patients with oropharyngeal carcinoma. *Head & Neck, 29*(11), 1024–1032. https://doi.org/10.1002/hed.20623
Rieger, J. M., Zalmanowitz, J. G., & Wolfaardt, J. F. (2006). Functional outcomes after organ preservation treatment in head and neck cancer: A critical review of the literature. *International Journal of Oral and Maxillofacial Surgery, 35*, 581–587.
Seikaly, H. (2008). Beavertail modification of the radial forearm free flap in base of tongue reconstruction: Technique and functional outcomes. *Head & Neck, 31*(2), 213–219. https://doi.org/10.1002/hed.20953
Seikaly, H., Rieger, J., Wolfaardt, J., Moysa, G., Harris, J., & Jha, N. (2003). Functional outcomes after primary oropharyngeal cancer resection and reconstruction with the radial forearm free flap. *The Laryngoscope, 113*(5), 897–904. https://doi.org/10.1097/00005537-200305000-00023
Shaw, D. W., Williams, R. B. H., Cook, I. J., Wallace, K. L., Weltman, M. D., Collins, P. J., … Simula, M. E. (2004). Oropharyngeal scintigraphy: A reliable technique for the quantitative evaluation of oral-pharyngeal swallowing. *Dysphagia, 19*(1), 36–42. https://doi.org/10.1007/s00455-003-0033-7
Shiboski, C. H., Schmidt, B. L., & Jordan, R. C. K. (2005). Tongue and tonsil carcinoma. *Cancer, 103*(9), 1843–1849. https://doi.org/10.1002/cncr.20998
Shin, Y. S., Koh, Y. W., Kim, S. H., Jeong, J. H., & Ahn, S. (2012). Radiotherapy deteriorates postoperative functional outcome after partial glossectomy with free flap reconstruction. *Journal of Oral and Maxillofacial Surgery, 70*, 216–220.
Siegel, R., Naishadham, D., & Jemal, A. (2013). Cancer statistics, 2013. *CA: A Cancer Journal for Clinicians, 63*(1), 11–30. https://doi.org/10.3322/caac.21166
Spiro, R. H., & Strong, E. W. (1974). Surgical treatment of cancer of the tongue. *The Surgical Clinics of North America, 54*(4), 759–765.
Stelzle, F., Knipfer, C., Schuster, M., & Bocklet, T. (2013). Factors influencing relative speech intelligibility in patients with oral squamous cell carcinoma: A prospective study using automatic, computer-based speech analysis. *Journal of Oral and Maxillofacial Surgery, 42*, 1377–1384.
Su, W. (2003). Functional comparison after reconstruction with a radial forearm free flap or a pectoralis major flap for cancer of the tongue. *Otolaryngology – Head and Neck Surgery, 128*(3), 412–418. https://doi.org/10.1067/mhn.2003.38
Suarez-Cunqueiro, M.-M., Schramm, A., Schoen, R., Seoane-Lestón, J., Otero-Cepeda, X.-L., Bormann, K.-H., … Gellrich, N. C. (2008). Speech and swallowing impairment after treatment for oral and oropharyngeal cancer. *Archives of Otolaryngology–Head & Neck Surgery, 134*(12), 1299–1304. https://doi.org/10.1001/archotol.134.12.1299
Sun, J., Weng, Y., Li, J., Wang, G., & Zhang, Z. (2007). Analysis of determinants on speech function after glossectomy. *Journal of Oral Maxillofacial Surgery, 65*(10), 1944–1950. https://doi.org/10.1016/j.joms.2006.11.017
Teichgraeber, J., Bowman, J., & Goepfert, H. (1985). New test series for the functional evaluation of oral cavity cancer. *Head & Neck Surgery, 8*(1), 9–20.

Thankappan, K., Kuriakose, M. A., Chatni, S. S., Sharan, R., Trivedi, N. P., Vijayaraghavan, S., … Iyer, S. (2011). Lateral arm free flap for oral tongue reconstruction. *Annals of Plastic Surgery, 66*(3), 261–266. https://doi.org/10.1097/SAP.0b013e3181d50e9e

Thoné, M., Karengera, D., Siciliano, S., & Reychler, H. (2003). Reconstruction of the mobile tongue malignant tumor excision: Quality-of-life assessment in 19 patients. *Revue de Stomatologie et de Chirurgie Maxillo-Faciale, 104*(1), 19–24.

Urken, M. L. (2003). Advances in head and neck reconstruction. *The Laryngoscope, 113*(9), 1473–1476. https://doi.org/10.1097/00005537-200309000-00008

Urken, M. L., & Biller, H. F. (1994). A new bilobed design for the sensate radial forearm flap to preserve tongue mobility following significant glossectomy. *Archives of Otolaryngology–Head & Neck Surgery, 120*(1), 26–31. https://doi.org/10.1001/archotol.1994.01880250022002

Urken, M. L., Moscoso, J. F., Lawson, W., & Biller, H. F. (1994). A systematic approach to functional reconstruction of the oral cavity following partial and total glossectomy. *Archives of Otolaryngology–Head & Neck Surgery, 120*(6), 589–601. https://doi.org/10.1001/archotol.1994.01880300007002

Uwiera, T., Seikaly, H., Rieger, J., Chau, J., & Harris, J. (2004). Functional outcomes after hemiglossectomy and reconstruction with a bilobed radial forearm free flap. *Journal of Otolaryngology, 33*(6), 356–359.

Warnakulasuriya, S. (2009). Global epidemiology of oral and oropharyngeal cancer. *Oral Oncology, 45*(4–5), 309–316. https://doi.org/10.1016/j.oraloncology.2008.06.002

Yu, P., & Robb, G. L. (2005). Reconstruction for total and near-total glossectomy defects. *Clinics in Plastic Surgery, 32*(3), 411–419. https://doi.org/10.1016/j.cps.2005.02.005

Yun, I. S., Lee, D. W., Lee, W. J., Lew, D. H., Choi, E. C., & Rah, D. K. (2010). Correlation of neotongue volume changes with functional outcomes after long-term follow-up of total glossectomy. *Journal of Craniofacial Surgery, 21*(1), 111–116. https://doi.org/10.1097/SCS.0b013e3181c46692

Zuydam, A. C., Lowe, D., Brown, J. S., Vaughan, E. D., & Rogers, S. N. (2005). Predictors of speech and swallowing function following primary surgery for oral and oropharyngeal cancer. *Clinical Otolaryngology, 30*(5), 428–437. https://doi.org/10.1111/j.1365-2273.2005.01061.x

Chapter 7
Psychosocial Considerations for Cancer Patients in a Pediatric Intensive Care Unit at a Large, Freestanding Children's Hospital

Mara L. Leimanis and Sandra K. Zuiderveen

Introduction

The prognosis for children with a cancer diagnosis has improved steadily over the last decades, with 5-year survival rates increasing from ~40% in the 1970s, and doubling to ~80% in the 2000s (Kaatsch, 2010; Steliarova-Foucher et al., 2004). In spite of the many different types of cancers that are diagnosed in children of different ages, their increased survival rates are likely due, in part, to advancements in cancer screening and prevention, treatment options, and life-prolonging support systems (e.g., extracorporeal membrane oxygenation [ECMO]). However, depending on the patient's age at diagnosis, the type of cancer, and the course of treatment, medical outcomes continue to vary greatly (Dursun et al., 2009).

This chapter describes the pediatric oncology patients of a high-volume tertiary care facility and includes a discussion of psychosocial concerns, environmental stressors, and communication practices related to pediatric cancer patients in the pediatric intensive care unit (PICU). Although concepts are presented within the context of a specific institution, we believe they may be relevant for health-care and oncology providers in any PICU setting. From this chapter the reader will be able to (a) describe the demographics of pediatric cancer patients as admitted to a freestanding, high-volume tertiary care children's hospital in an urban setting, (b) describe two forms of communication that take place in a PICU, (c) identify some key environmental stressors and themes of involuntary exposure to trauma leading to distress, and (d) critique the psychosocial implications of these factors for the patient and the family, including peri-traumatic dissociation.

A pediatric cancer population is heterogeneous in nature and challenging to treat given the rapidly developing biology of the child and changing psychosocial needs of the family (Wiener, Hersh, & Alderfer, 2011) (for the purposes of this chapter, the

M. L. Leimanis (✉) · S. K. Zuiderveen
Pediatric Critical Care, Helen DeVos Children's Hospital, Grand Rapids, MI, USA
e-mail: Mara.Leimanis@spectrumhealth.org

T. R. Fitzpatrick (ed.), *Quality of Life Among Cancer Survivors*,
https://doi.org/10.1007/978-3-319-75223-5_7

term "family" includes designated caregivers). In addition to the immediate challenges surrounding a hospitalization, communication issues between the family and the clinical care team can quickly arise. Physical and physiological stressors of the illness are compounded with parents/guardians who are left to navigate unfamiliar and intimidating hospital settings. In certain instances, transition from a pediatric oncology unit to a PICU may be necessary and unexpected, potentially compounding the stress (Demaret, Pettersen, Hubert, Teira, & Emeriaud, 2012).

Although the topic of pediatric oncology has been explored extensively in medical terms (Fisher & Rheingold, 2011), there are few prospective studies regarding the PICU oncology experience and the specific challenges that result from working with this vulnerable population, which this chapter will not address specifically (Howell, Kutko, & Greenwald, 2011). Effectively managing the PICU course of oncology patients includes pain management, child-life services, and consultations with other sub-disciplines. In particular, transitions in care from a pediatric oncology unit to a PICU need to include wide-ranging clinical decisions and the consideration of environmental stressors (e.g., alarms and noises, such as crying and conversations, light exposure, air quality) and restrictions on family members in a more tightly regulated hospital environment.

As provisions of care evolve, hospitals are increasingly attentive to these environmental factors and the milieu in which care is provided. Concerns about patient satisfaction, psychological distress, coping skills, and quality of life are receiving increased attention and being integrated into the daily care of patients. The burdens of patient and family stress in both pediatric oncology units and PICUs can be alleviated by the involvement of the entire clinical care team, which is often large (>10 individuals) and can include oncologists, nurses, nurse practitioners, intensive care specialists, dietitians, respiratory therapists, social workers, chaplains, pain and palliative care specialists, other medical specialists, child-life specialists, and clinical ethicists.

Overview: Pediatric Cancer Patients

To begin, it is important to note that the definition of the term "pediatric cancer patient" includes not only the child involved, but family members as caregivers and legal guardians of that child. Consent for children's care is provided by the parents/guardians until the age of "assent" in children, which is approximately 7–11 years old. In this age group, children who are deemed of minimal cognitive age to provide consent may also be included in the decision-making process (Dorn, Susman, & Fletcher, 1995). Ultimately, the parent/guardian remains responsible for consent to procedures (including drug regimens) for their child. This is relevant because the family unit can include two or more individuals (i.e. child-patient, and parent/guardian), all of whose opinions need to be considered.

Pediatric cancers are generally defined as those affecting children up to the age of 18. However, in some instances, patients past the age of 18 retain their relationship with their pediatric oncologist and may return to their pediatric hospital for further care and long-term follow-up. Patients may continue to utilize the treatment protocols related to their pediatric cancers up to the age of 26, on a case-by-case basis (Freyer & Brugieres, 2008). They may require medical attention for long-term health issues that resulted from their pediatric cancer treatments as now adult survivors (Lipshultz et al., 2014; Oeffinger et al., 2006; Tukenova et al., 2010). This is an area that requires further investigation.

Historically, pediatric oncology patients were cared for within an adult hospital setting according to the procedures and policies of an existing hospital framework; practitioners frequently adapted methods used to treat adults for their pediatric patients (DeVita & Chu, 2008). With the development and expansion of specialized children's hospitals (such as St. Jude, est. 1962), there has been an evolution in the way cancer patients are treated in an inpatient setting, particularly in relation to the application of pediatric-specific quality and safety standards (Neuss et al., 2017). Accomplishing this has required hospital administrators, clinical care providers, and the community to champion the delivery of specialized care for children. The development of freestanding children's hospitals distinct from the adult setting has further allowed health-care facilities to customize and tailor their approach to the medical and psychosocial needs of all children, including the youngest cancer patients (Fisher et al., 2014).

This customized children's hospital environment can prove to be especially important for pediatric oncology patients, consisting largely of children with neurological, hematological, head, neck, bone, or tissue cancers. Cancer patients with an acutely worsening condition may require the attention of an intensive care facility, as is required in up to 38% of children (Rosenman, Vik, Hui, & Breitfeld, 2005). Given that the 5-year survival rate is now up to 83% for children's cancers, a PICU transfer is often required and may be part of the patient treatment trajectory (Rosenman et al., 2005).

Various severity of illness scores are used to measure patient acuity. This score is measured in pediatric patients early in their PICU admission—typically during the first 12 h—before any influence of therapy. One of these acuity measures is the Pediatric Risk of Mortality (PRISM) score, which correlates the physiologic status with risk of mortality (M. M. Pollack, Ruttimann, & Getson, 1988). This scoring system has evolved over the years; it is now in its third iteration and readily used in most PICUs (Pollack, Patel, & Ruttimann, 1996).

It should be noted that the PRISM score was further developed in 2000 specifically for oncology, which led to the acronym "O" for oncology in "O-PRISM." This refinement of the scoring system stemmed from some debate regarding the validity of the PRISM score for oncology patients and its later development. It was found to more accurately predict the mortality in ICU bone marrow transplant patients (Schneider et al., 2000) and event-free survival. A high O-PRISM score at the time of admission was predictive of a poorer long-term outcome (Fernandez-Garcia, Gonzalez-Vicent, Mastro-Martinez, Serrano, & Diaz, 2015).

In a recent study reviewing 5 years of patients in a developing country, sepsis and respiratory failure were reported as the most frequent reasons for PICU admissions, requiring urgent intervention with inotropic support, oxygen therapy, and mechanical ventilation (Ali, Sayed, & Mohammed, 2016). In this developing hospital setting, these factors were associated with poor outcomes, especially for those patients with hematological malignancies. In another study, by Dursun et al. (2009) in a Turkish PICU population, risk factors included the number of organ system dysfunctions ($n > 2$), sepsis, the need for mechanical ventilation, positive inotropic support, and high PRISM III scores (>10) which were negatively associated with survival.

Clinical factors can be exacerbated by the human factor. Pediatric oncology patients who are transferred or sent to a PICU may encounter a situation where the clinical staff are limited in their ability to offer treatment to the patient, especially in the case of a terminal diagnosis. A quote by Theodore Roosevelt conveys the danger inherent in aggressive therapeutic approaches when faced with the bleakest of prognoses: "optimism is a good characteristic but if carried to excess, becomes foolishness" (Peters & Agbeko, 2014) p. 1589). This can be seen in the determination of an oncologist attempting to give a patient one last round of chemotherapy. There are instances when palliative chemotherapy is considered, but can lead to needless prolonging of life and suffering. The question then becomes: when to stop therapeutic interventional treatments and transition to supportive care?

Generally, this can cause a certain degree of nihilism and can be a challenging time for the clinical staff (Christakis & Asch, 1995; Cook et al., 1995; Randolph, Zollo, Wigton, & Yeh, 1997). In one cross-sectional study that surveyed 56 caregivers, 7 patient characteristics were described as the most important factors influencing decisions specifically, family preferences (76%), probability of survival (50%), and functional status (47%) were listed in the top three (Randolph et al., 1997). Evidence from other studies provides insight into the process influencing caregiver decision-making with the use of algorithms (Demaret et al., 2012), which includes family preferences. Oncology patients in a PICU setting will now be discussed.

PICU Oncology Patients of a High-Volume Tertiary Care Facility

To explore the psychosocial and communication issues, and environmental stressors related to cancer patients and PICUs, it is helpful to have an example—in this case, a modern, urban, high-volume pediatric tertiary care facility in Western Michigan.

Helen DeVos Children's Hospital (HDVCH) is located in Grand Rapids, Michigan. HDVCH operates under the umbrella of Spectrum Health Hospital System, which includes three hospitals in Grand Rapids and nine regional hospitals serving patients across all of Western and Northern Michigan. HDVCH was created at Spectrum Health in 1993 to fill a critical need for a tertiary care referral center devoted to infants, children, and adolescents in the area; in January 2011 HDVCH moved to a newly built, freestanding, 11-story facility (Connors, 2010). HDVCH has a separate PICU on the 8th floor, which handles more than 1500 admissions and 6000 patient days per year. Seventeen board certified intensivists cover the unit, caring for up to 36 critically ill children, with extra patient beds on the 7th floor.

For the purpose of this chapter, and to better understand the patient demographics of PICU oncology patients at HDVCH, we pulled all local patient admissions with an oncological diagnosis ($N = 187$) from January 2012 to December 2015 from a pediatric critical care registry: Virtual Pediatric Intensive Care Unit Performance Systems (VPS, LLC, Los Angeles, CA). Our assumption was, that the reason for admission and cancer type, might influence the length of stay (LOS) and provide some insight into the psychosocial implications for care.

VPS was established in 2006 to create a cohesive and definitive central capture mechanism for data from all PICUs. It is now an international registry with 135 participating hospitals and >1,000,000 PICU cases, which provides accurate and representative local data, collected daily by site coordinators, and reported through the Clinical Program Performance Reports for Pediatric Critical Care (Wetzel, Sachedeva, & Rice, 2011). Spectrum Health Internal Review Board (IRB) approval was not obtained for this research, as only a minimal, de-identified data set was retrieved; it included age at admission, LOS in the PICU, race/ethnicity, sex, primary and secondary reason(s) for admission, cancer diagnosis, and included perioperative patients.

The resulting patient demographics are described in Table 7.1. The mean age of HDVCH PICU patients with an oncology diagnosis at admission was 114.9 months

Table 7.1 Patient demographics of total PICU admissions for 2012–2015 with an oncology diagnosis ($N = 187$)

	Range	(*n*)	%	Mean	[95% CI]	SD
Age (months)						
6–275				114.9	104.9–125.0	69.5
Gender						
Male		122	65.2			
Female		65	34.8			
PICU LOS[a] (days)	0.3–53.8	187	100	4.7	3.7–5.7	7.0
Bone, tissue cancer	0.3–12.8	21	11.2	3.1	1.6–4.6	3.3
Hematological	0.4–25.5	51	27.3	4.1	2.6–5.5	5.2
Neurological	0.5–53.8	100	53.5	5.7	3.9–7.4	8.6
Ethnicity						
Caucasian/European		142	75.9			
Hispanic		23	12.3			
Other/mixed		9	4.8			
African-American		5	2.7			
Asian/Indian/Pacific		4	2.1			
Unspecified		4	2.1			

LOS length of stay, *PICU* pediatric intensive care unit

[a]One way analysis of variance, $p = 0.337$; due to the non-normal distribution of the data, values were log transformed prior to analysis; values in the table represent the actual data

(~ 9.5 years), with a range from 0.5 to 23 years of age. The demographics of patients admitted exceeded the customary age of 18 because some patients were treated as young adults with pediatric cancers, and their appropriate treatment course had been continued at the original diagnosis and treatment hospital. The dominance of a Caucasian/European ethnicity (75.9%) was in line with the general population demographics of the West Michigan region ("Population and Demographics," 2016). The neurological patients had the longest overall tendency for LOS as compared to bone/tissue (3.1 days) and hematological (4.1 days) with a mean of 5.7 days, before a patient was sent to another pediatric unit.

Table 7.2 describes the diagnoses for the admitted population of 187 patients. Neurological cancers made up more than half of the total diagnoses, with hematological cancers approximately another quarter of the population, followed by bone and tissue cancers. Neurological cancers made up the majority of admissions as these were surgical in nature (e.g., tumor resection/removal, biopsy retrieval).

Just over half of the HDVCH PICU patients were admitted due to their cancer diagnosis. As Table 7.3 shows, 48.1% presented with an acute symptom due to an underlying cancer diagnosis, such as infections, neurological issues, or cardiovascular/circulatory symptoms.

Psychosocial Issues

For pediatric cancer patients like those at HDVCH, a PICU, by definition, provides a higher level of care and offers "one-on-one" patient-nursing capacity, if needed. This allows the patient to be the sole focus and receive more intensive, focused care. One way in which a PICU differs from a hospital oncology unit is that it enforces greater restrictions on the patient as well as the family. These can include limitations in visiting hours and/or the numbers and types of visitor allowed (e.g., parent/guardian only). There may also be limitations on the physical proximity permitted between the parent/guardian and the child, due to the presence of tubing and/or ventilators. These physical restrictions may interfere with the child's mobility and/or limit the ability of the parent/guardian to be close to them (e.g., intubated children), resulting in an increase in parental stress levels (Aamir, Mittal, Kaushik, Kashyap, & Kaur, 2014).

Additional stressors to the family can include the introduction of new clinical staff to the family. Patients may have built a relationship with their oncologist, and now their previous physician has ceded care to the intensivist in the PICU. Although an oncology nurse may remain present for continuity of care, this can be a stressful time for the patient and the family as they are introduced to a new environment and new care team. Combined, all of this can generate a "perfect storm" for the parents/guardians, creating what has been termed peri-traumatic dissociation—defined as a state of limited or distorted awareness during and immediately after a stressful event (Bronner et al., 2009; Marmar, Weiss, & Metzler, 1997).

Table 7.2 Summary of oncological diagnoses of total PICU admissions for 2012–2015 ($N = 187$)

Groups	(n)	%
Bone, tissue cancer	21	11.2
Rhabdomyosarcoma	2	1.1
+ Secondary malignancies	1	0.5
+ Pharynx neoplasm	1	0.5
Osteosarcoma	4	2.1
Ewing sarcoma	11	5.9
+ Lung neoplasm	4	2.1
+ Brain neoplasm	1	0.5
Cartilage neoplasm	1	0.5
Head and neck	5	2.7
Middle ear neoplasm	1	0.5
Nasopharyngeal	1	0.5
Thymus neoplasm	3	1.6
Hematological	51	27.3
Acute lymphoid leukemia	36	19.2
Acute myeloid leukemia	5	2.7
Burkitt's lymphoma	4	2.1
Hodgkin's lymphoma	5	2.7
Non-Hodgkins lymphoma	1	0.5
Neurological	100	53.5
Astrocytoma	21	11.2
Brain neoplasm (unspecified)	39	20.9
Craniopharyngioma	3	1.6
Glioma	3	1.6
Medulloblastoma	8	4.3
Neuroblastoma	17	9.1
+ Peritoneum/colon neoplasm	1	0.5
+ Endocrine gland neoplasm	1	0.5
Neuroendocrine carcinoma adenoma	2	1.1
Spinal cord neoplasm	2	1.1
Reproductive: female genital organ neoplasm	3	1.6
Other organs	7	3.7
Liver neoplasms	1	0.5
Pelvis/trunk neoplasm	2	1.1
Germinoma	1	0.5
Endocrine gland neoplasm	3	1.6

PICU pediatric intensive care unit

Psychosocial issues in pediatric cancers are complex, dynamic, and multidimensional. The family unit includes not just parents/guardians but the siblings, other family members, the larger family system, and the immediate community. Depending on the age of the child at the time of diagnosis, a range of events can take place, which can include disruptions in social development (Katz, Rubinstein,

Table 7.3 Primary reasons for admission to the PICU for patients from 2012 to 2015 with an oncology diagnosis ($N = 187$)

	(*n*)	%[a]
PICU admission due to cancer	98	51.9
1° cancer	97	51.3
2° cancers	1	0.53
PICU admission due to other symptoms	91	48.1
Infections	29	15.3
Sepsis with or without shock	18	9.52
Influenza (varia, viral)	4	2.1
Bacterial (pneumonia, septicemia)	7	3.7
Neurological	27	14.3
Convulsions/seizures	6	3.2
Altered mental status	4	2.1
Cerebral thrombosis	4	2.1
Encephalopathy	5	2.6
Hydrocephalus	3	1.6
Intracranial hemorrhage	3	1.6
Other	1	0.5
Cardiovascular/circulatory	20	10.6
Atrial fibrillation	2	1.1
Pulmonary insufficiency	10	5.3
Pericardial effusion	4	2.1
Hypovolemic shock/dehydration	3	1.6
Respiratory arrest	1	0.5
Hematological	4	2.1
Neutropenia	3	1.6
TRALI	1	0.5
Renal	2	1.1
Other	9	4.8
Chronic disease of tonsils/adenoids	1	0.5
Peritonitis	1	0.5
Complications varia	6	3.2
Surgical complications	1	0.5

LOS length of stay, *PICU* pediatric intensive care unit, *TRALI* transfusion-related acute lung injury

Note: [a] Percentages may not add up to 100% due to missing data

Hubert, & Blew, 1989), absences from school (Cairns, Klopovich, Hearne, & Lansky, 1982), and disruptions in family dynamics (Brody & Simmons, 2007). Long-term side effects of treatments and medications can persist for some time, with fatigue being reported as the most critical factor in the transition back to school and daily life (Clarke-Steffen, 2001; Hockenberry-Eaton & Hinds, 2000). In addition, a pediatric cancer diagnosis can negatively affect the parent/guardian, resulting in adverse health effects after a PICU admission, with an increased tendency toward suicide, absences from work, and reports of post-traumatic stress disorder (PTSD) for both the parent/guardian (Balluffi et al., 2004), and the child (Rees, Gledhill, Garralda, & Nadel, 2004). Lastly, financial burdens can ensue with mounting medical expenses (for a systematic literature review, see Shudy et al. 2006).

Communication

Communication practices related to pediatric cancer patients in the PICU can be broken down into a few different frameworks. There is parent/child communication, which we do not address in this chapter. There is also the communication that happens with the family or "family-centered communication." And there is cooperative communication, which is communication that takes place between care providers and the family but bypasses any perceived hierarchical structures.

Family-centered communication includes practitioner/family interactions, typically in the form of daily bedside rounds, which take place between 8 a.m. and 11 a.m. Rounds allow the family to meet with the clinical care team and obtain accumulative information regarding their child's condition and treatment plan for the day(s). Families at this time are encouraged to ask questions and participate in the dialogue. The information is compressed and passed on to the family within a 15–30-min timeframe. This method of communication has developed from theoretical models from a PICU setting—encouraging cross talk, family engagement, and communication with clinical experts—during which the entire clinical team may be present (Baird, Davies, Hinds, Baggott, & Rehm, 2015). This communication comes at a time when the family will feel a sense of disruption, disappointment, and anxiety in the PICU environment, experience a loss of control and yet still desire a continuity of care for their child (Baird, Rehm, Hinds, Baggott, & Davies, 2016; Haggerty et al., 2003).

Specifically, Haggerty et al. describes the term "relational continuity", as trust building over time between patients/families and individual care providers. The importance of communications about patient care cannot be overestimated, as frustration, hyper-vigilance, and mistrust can be avoided and lessened with effective communication practices (Epstein, Miles, Rovnyak, & Baernholdt, 2013; Heller, Solomon, & Initiative for Pediatric Palliative Care Investigator, 2005). Continuity of care promoted by effective communication has been shown to positively affect patient outcomes and lead to fewer nurse-related adverse events (Siow, Wypij, Berry, Hickey, & Curley, 2013). In one investigation of parental satisfaction, a network analysis was employed, which found that the care team's structure was more important than its size (Gray et al., 2010).

Communication that takes place between couples, clinical staff, and care providers in a given department within a hospital, or between families and care providers, is termed "cooperative communication." This form of communication may also occur with siblings and the extended family members (the opposite of which is termed confrontational communication). Cooperative communication is a form of communication that is encouraged for families and the clinical care team, also termed parallel communication (Kamihara, Nyborn, Olcese, Nickerson, & Mack, 2015). This can help move a family away from secrecy and collusion and promote positive discourse. In another context, enhancing and encouraging cooperative communication has been shown to be effective for families and nursing home staff, promoting trust and improving family-staff relations at an otherwise stressful time (Pillemer et al., 2003). This results in improved attitudes, the ability to work better together, families reporting less conflict with staff, and staff reporting a decreased likelihood of quitting their jobs, so all in all positive.

Environmental Stressors

When a pediatric cancer patient transfers to a PICU from a pediatric oncology unit, this transition can be sudden, unexpected, and fraught with fear and stress for the family (Khanna, Finlay, Jatana, Gouffe, & Redshaw, 2016). In the most extreme cases, the family may not even be present when the transfer happens; they may be absent due to work (or other). Communication among the clinical staff will also be in transition, as staff from both units must rapidly communicate, understand, and adapt to the complex medical needs of the newly arrived PICU patient. They may have limited time in an acute situation to communicate with family members.

Once a patient is admitted to a PICU, there is a change in the immediate environment for both the patient and the family. If the patient was previously on a pediatric oncology floor, there may have been familiarity with the staff, a sense of routine, and certain privileges or freedoms available to friends and family, depending on the medical condition of the patient. In the PICU, the intensity of care is increased and restricted, as mentioned previously (e.g., tests may need to be administered at designated times instead of at the convenience of the patient or family). The use of strong lighting and alarms may be an irritant, along with not being able to coordinate care around the normal circadian rhythms of the patient. Unit-based rules profoundly affect both the patient and the family (Baird et al., 2015), however, are necessary for this chaotic, unpredictable, noisy environment and with so many different care providers, as described in the introduction (Clarke, 2005).

The work of Khanna et al. (2016) showed that involuntary exposure to observed trauma in the PICU was a source of distress and included a few main themes: (a) seeing and hearing people crying, (b) the deterioration and/or appearance of another patient, and (c) seeing children/parents in distress. Other themes included the absence of privacy and confidentiality, insufficient empathy for children and their families, the need for personal reflection and growth, and staff communication. The involuntary environmental exposures were defined as overhearing family members' conversations, crying, alarms, witnessing seizures, cardiopulmonary resuscitation, or death, all of which did not necessarily involve their own child. Collectively, these exposures were a great source of distress that could potentially be alleviated with short-term supports.

Perhaps the greatest environmental distress for the family occurs when a child is in isolation in a PICU. All visitors, including parents/guardians, must wear a gown, gloves, and/or a mask when indicated to prevent the inadvertent exposure and transmission of an outside infection to the patient. Guidelines for appropriate procedures are defined by the national Centers for Disease Control and Prevention (CDC), as described in Mehta et al. (Mehta et al., 2014).

Suggested visitation guidelines at HDVCH have attempted to address some of these issues in an effort to minimize environmental stressors to the patient and staff. These include, but are not limited to, reduced visiting hours for siblings, relatives, and friends, no visitors during shift changes (7 a.m.–8 a.m. and 7 p.m.–8 p.m.), only two people allowed to stay overnight at the child's bedside, and no more than three people at the patient's bedside at any one time, based on the child's condition. In addition, families are encouraged to keep personal belongings in the family space, and hand washing is encouraged for everyone going into and out of the room. In certain instances, when the patient is best served by being kept in a low-stimulation room (e.g., the sedated-mechanically-ventilated child), it is recommended that low volumes, dim lights, and a careful, caring touch are administered.

Implications for Clinical Practice

Studies have shown that up to 38% of pediatric oncology patients will require PICU admission within 3 years of diagnosis, with a mortality rate of 6.8% which is almost three times higher than the general PICU population (2.4%) (Zinter, DuBois, Spicer, Matthay, & Sapru, 2014). Hematological cancer patients have the greatest PICU admission acuity, rates of infection, and mortality compared to those with solid tumors, according to Zinter et al. In our patient population, infection also contributed to PICU admissions. It can be challenging to describe, in advance, the changing and evolving needs of these children. There is a desire to maintain relational continuity (as previously defined by Haggerty et. al. in the Communication section) among the patients, families, and individual care providers, as has been described for parents of children with severe disabilities (Graham, Pemstein, & Curley, 2009) and for those that are technology-dependent (Reeves, Timmons, & Dampier, 2006). Unfortunately, relational continuity is not necessarily an integral part of routine care, as discussed by Baird et al. 2016.

One potential barrier to achieving this relational continuity in a PICU setting may be the working preferences of nurses, who might desire to continue caring for a diverse patient population in the PICU and who also may attempt to minimize emotional entanglement with oncology patients (Baird et al., 2016). In this compelling article, Baird describes the following implications in the continuity of nursing care: "nurses understood the need but faced both contextual and personal challenges to achieving continuity, including fluctuations in staffing needs, training demands, fear of emotional entanglement, and concern for missed learning opportunities (p. 1)."

Utilizing cooperative communication in a fluid, ongoing manner, it is possible to prepare the family ahead of time for the potential that a PICU admission may be necessary and thereby decrease stress for the family. Once patients are approximately 7 years old or older, they may become more involved with this cooperative communication. This is especially important for the adolescent and the young adult populations and further investigation is required into their specific psychosocial needs (Straehla et al., 2017).

We believe research in the area of the pediatric PICU experience has significant clinical implications and the potential to lead to best practices for both the developed and the developing world regarding incidence, survival and care, and further implications for psychosocial interventions (Ali et al., 2016). Evolution of this work will result in better interventions and potentiate coping strategies to negate some of the stressful effects and events surrounding a cancer diagnosis and PICU admission in the youngest and most vulnerable of populations.

Acknowledgments VPS data was provided by Virtual Pediatric Systems, LLC. No endorsement or editorial restriction of the interpretation of these data or opinions of the authors has been implied or stated.

The authors would like to thank Dawn Eding, RN; Craig Vandellen, MSW; Dr. Deanna Mitchell; Dr. Surender Rajasekaran; and Dr. Rick Hackbarth, as well as the clinical oncology and PICU staff at Helen DeVos Children's Hospital, for their support in the completion of this chapter and various contributions.

The authors would also like to thank Beyond Words, Inc., for assistance with the editing and preparation of this manuscript. The authors maintained control over the direction and content of this article during its development. Although Beyond Words, Inc., supplied professional editing services, this does not indicate its endorsement of, agreement with, or responsibility for the content of the article.

Conflicts of Interest The authors have no conflicts of interest or funding sources to declare.

Disclaimer The opinions and views expressed in this chapter do not in any way reflect the views of Helen DeVos Children's Hospital, other sites of Spectrum Health, other sites affiliated with Helen DeVos Children's Hospital or Spectrum Health, or the staff employed by Helen DeVos Children's Hospital, Spectrum Health, or any affiliated members.

References

Aamir, M., Mittal, K., Kaushik, J. S., Kashyap, H., & Kaur, G. (2014). Predictors of stress among parents in pediatric intensive care unit: A prospective observational study. *Indian Journal of Pediatrics*, *81*(11), 1167–1170. https://doi.org/10.1007/s12098-014-1415-6

Ali, A. M., Sayed, H. A., & Mohammed, M. M. (2016). The outcome of critically ill pediatric cancer patients admitted to the pediatric intensive care unit in a tertiary university oncology Center in a Developing Country: A 5-year experience. *Journal of Pediatric Hematology/Oncology*, *38*(5), 355–359. https://doi.org/10.1097/MPH.0000000000000523

Baird, J., Davies, B., Hinds, P. S., Baggott, C., & Rehm, R. S. (2015). What impact do hospital and unit-based rules have upon patient and family-centered care in the pediatric intensive care unit? *Journal of Pediatric Nursing*, *30*(1), 133–142. https://doi.org/10.1016/j.pedn.2014.10.001

Baird, J., Rehm, R. S., Hinds, P. S., Baggott, C., & Davies, B. (2016). Do you know my child? Continuity of nursing Care in the Pediatric Intensive Care Unit. *Nursing Research, 65*(2), 142–150. https://doi.org/10.1097/NNR.0000000000000135

Balluffi, A., Kassam-Adams, N., Kazak, A., Tucker, M., Dominguez, T., & Helfaer, M. (2004). Traumatic stress in parents of children admitted to the pediatric intensive care unit. *Pediatric Critical Care Medicine, 5*(6), 547–553. https://doi.org/10.1097/01.PCC.0000137354.19807.44

Brody, A. C., & Simmons, L. A. (2007). Family resiliency during childhood cancer: The father's perspective. *Journal of Pediatric Oncology Nursing, 24*(3), 152–165. https://doi.org/10.1177/1043454206298844

Bronner, M. B., Kayser, A. M., Knoester, H., Bos, A. P., Last, B. F., & Grootenhuis, M. A. (2009). A pilot study on peritraumatic dissociation and coping styles as risk factors for posttraumatic stress, anxiety and depression in parents after their child's unexpected admission to a Pediatric Intensive Care Unit. *Child Adolesc Psychiatry Ment Health, 3*(1), 33. https://doi.org/10.1186/1753-2000-3-33

Cairns, N. U., Klopovich, P., Hearne, E., & Lansky, S. B. (1982). School attendance of children with cancer. *The Journal of School Health, 52*(3), 152–155. Retrieved from http://www.ncbi.nlm.nih.gov/pubmed/6916955.

Christakis, N. A., & Asch, D. A. (1995). Physician characteristics associated with decisions to withdraw life support. *American Journal of Public Health, 85*(3), 367–372. Retrieved from http://www.ncbi.nlm.nih.gov/pubmed/7892921

Clarke, A. (2005). *Situational analysis: Grounded theory after the postmodern turn*. Thousand Oaks, CA: Sage Publications.

Clarke-Steffen, L. (2001). Cancer-related fatigue in children. *Journal of Pediatric Oncology Nursing, 18*(2 Suppl 1), 1–2. Retrieved from http://www.ncbi.nlm.nih.gov/pubmed/11321844

Connors, R. Helen DeVos Children's Hospital. (2010). Inaugural Speech, Opening of Helen DeVos Children's Hospital [Press release]

Cook, D. J., Guyatt, G. H., Jaeschke, R., Reeve, J., Spanier, A., King, D., ... Streiner, D. L. (1995). Determinants in Canadian health care workers of the decision to withdraw life support from the critically ill. Canadian Critical Care Trials Group. *JAMA, 273*(9), 703–708. Retrieved from http://www.ncbi.nlm.nih.gov/pubmed/7853627

Demaret, P., Pettersen, G., Hubert, P., Teira, P., & Emeriaud, G. (2012). The critically-ill pediatric hemato-oncology patient: Epidemiology, management, and strategy of transfer to the pediatric intensive care unit. *Annals of Intensive Care, 2*(1), 14. https://doi.org/10.1186/2110-5820-2-14

DeVita, V. T., & Chu, E. (2008). A history of cancer chemotherapy. *Cancer Research, 68*(21), 8643–8653. https://doi.org/10.1158/0008-5472.CAN-07-6611

Dorn, L. D., Susman, E. J., & Fletcher, J. C. (1995). Informed consent in children and adolescents: Age, maturation and psychological state. *The Journal of Adolescent Health, 16*(3), 185–190. https://doi.org/10.1016/1054-139X(94)00063-K

Dursun, O., Hazar, V., Karasu, G. T., Uygun, V., Tosun, O., & Yesilipek, A. (2009). Prognostic factors in pediatric cancer patients admitted to the pediatric intensive care unit. *Journal of Pediatric Hematology/Oncology, 31*(7), 481–484. https://doi.org/10.1097/MPH.0b013e3181a330ef

Epstein, E. G., Miles, A., Rovnyak, V., & Baernholdt, M. (2013). Parents' perceptions of continuity of care in the neonatal intensive care unit: Pilot testing an instrument and implications for the nurse-parent relationship. *The Journal of Perinatal & Neonatal Nursing, 27*(2), 168–175. https://doi.org/10.1097/JPN.0b013e31828eafbb

Fernandez-Garcia, M., Gonzalez-Vicent, M., Mastro-Martinez, I., Serrano, A., & Diaz, M. A. (2015). Intensive care unit admissions among children after hematopoietic stem cell transplantation: Incidence, outcome, and prognostic factors. *Journal of Pediatric Hematology/Oncology, 37*(7), 529–535. https://doi.org/10.1097/MPH.0000000000000401

Fisher, B. T., Harris, T., Torp, K., Seif, A. E., Shah, A., Huang, Y. S., ... Aplenc, R. (2014). Establishment of an 11-year cohort of 8733 pediatric patients hospitalized at United States free-standing children's hospitals with de novo acute lymphoblastic leukemia from health care administrative data. *Medical Care, 52*(1), e1–e6. https://doi.org/10.1097/MLR.0b013e31824deff9

Fisher, M. J., & Rheingold, S. R. (2011). Oncologic emergencies. In P. Pizzo & D. Poplack (Eds.), *Principles and practice of pediatric oncology* (6th ed., pp. 1125–1151). Philadelphia, PA: Lippincott Williams and Wilkins.

Freyer, D. R., & Brugieres, L. (2008). Adolescent and young adult oncology: Transition of care. *Pediatric Blood & Cancer, 50*(5 Suppl), 1116–1119. https://doi.org/10.1002/pbc.21455

Graham, R. J., Pemstein, D. M., & Curley, M. A. (2009). Experiencing the pediatric intensive care unit: Perspective from parents of children with severe antecedent disabilities. *Critical Care Medicine, 37*(6), 2064–2070. https://doi.org/10.1097/CCM.0b013e3181a00578

Gray, J. E., Davis, D. A., Pursley, D. M., Smallcomb, J. E., Geva, A., & Chawla, N. V. (2010). Network analysis of team structure in the neonatal intensive care unit. *Pediatrics, 125*(6), e1460–e1467. https://doi.org/10.1542/peds.2009-2621

Haggerty, J. L., Reid, R. J., Freeman, G. K., Starfield, B. H., Adair, C. E., & McKendry, R. (2003). Continuity of care: A multidisciplinary review. *BMJ, 327*(7425), 1219–1221. https://doi.org/10.1136/bmj.327.7425.1219

Heller, K. S., Solomon, M. Z., & Initiative for Pediatric Palliative Care Investigator, T. (2005). Continuity of care and caring: What matters to parents of children with life-threatening conditions. *Journal of Pediatric Nursing, 20*(5), 335–346. https://doi.org/10.1016/j.pedn.2005.03.005

Hockenberry-Eaton, M., & Hinds, P. S. (2000). Fatigue in children and adolescents with cancer: Evolution of a program of study. *Seminars in Oncology Nursing, 16*(4), 261–272. discussion 272–268. Retrieved from http://www.ncbi.nlm.nih.gov/pubmed/11109271

Howell, J. D., Kutko, M. C., & Greenwald, B. M. (2011). Oncology patients in the pediatric intensive care unit: it's time for prospective study. *Pediatric Critical Care Medicine, 12*(6), 680–681. https://doi.org/10.1097/PCC.0b013e3182196cc2

Kaatsch, P. (2010). Epidemiology of childhood cancer. *Cancer Treatment Reviews, 36*(4), 277–285. https://doi.org/10.1016/j.ctrv.2010.02.003

Kamihara, J., Nyborn, J. A., Olcese, M. E., Nickerson, T., & Mack, J. W. (2015). Parental hope for children with advanced cancer. *Pediatrics, 135*(5), 868–874. https://doi.org/10.1542/peds.2014-2855

Katz, E., Rubinstein, C. L., Hubert, N. C., & Blew, A. (1989). School and social reintegration of children with cancer. *Journal of Psychosocial Oncology, 6*(3–4), 123–140.

Khanna, S., Finlay, J. K., Jatana, V., Gouffe, A. M., & Redshaw, S. (2016). The impact of observed trauma on parents in a PICU. *Pediatric Critical Care Medicine, 17*(4), e154–e158. https://doi.org/10.1097/PCC.0000000000000665

Lipshultz, S. E., Karnik, R., Sambatakos, P., Franco, V. I., Ross, S. W., & Miller, T. L. (2014). Anthracycline-related cardiotoxicity in childhood cancer survivors. *Current Opinion in Cardiology, 29*(1), 103–112. https://doi.org/10.1097/HCO.0000000000000034

Marmar, C. R., Weiss, D. S., & Metzler, T. J. (1997). In J. P. Wilson & T. M. Keane (Eds.), *The Peritraumatic dissociative experiences questionnaire. Assessing psychological trauma and PTSD: A handbook for practitioners*. New York, NY: The Guilford Press.

Mehta, Y., Gupta, A., Todi, S., Myatra, S., Samaddar, D. P., Patil, V., … Ramasubban, S. (2014). Guidelines for prevention of hospital acquired infections. *Indian Journal of Critical Care Medicine, 18*(3), 149–163. https://doi.org/10.4103/0972-5229.128705

Neuss, M. N., Gilmore, T. R., Belderson, K. M., Billett, A. L., Conti-Kalchik, T., Harvet, B. E., … Polovich, M. (2017). 2016 updated American Society of Clinical Oncology/Oncology Nursing Society chemotherapy administration safety standards, including standards for pediatric oncology. *Oncology Nursing Forum, 44*(1), 31–43. https://doi.org/10.1188/17.ONF.31-43

Oeffinger, K. C., Mertens, A. C., Sklar, C. A., Kawashima, T., Hudson, M. M., Meadows, A. T., … Childhood Cancer Survivor, S. (2006). Chronic health conditions in adult survivors of childhood cancer. *The New England Journal of Medicine, 355*(15), 1572–1582. https://doi.org/10.1056/NEJMsa060185

Peters, M. J., & Agbeko, R. S. (2014). Optimism and no longer foolishness? Haematology/oncology and the PICU. *Intensive Care Medicine, 40*(10), 1589–1591. https://doi.org/10.1007/s00134-014-3478-2

Pillemer, K., Suitor, J. J., Henderson, C. R., Jr., Meador, R., Schultz, L., Robison, J., & Hegeman, C. (2003). A cooperative communication intervention for nursing home staff and family members of residents. *Gerontologist, 43*(Spec No 2), 96–106. Retrieved from http://www.ncbi.nlm.nih.gov/pubmed/12711730

Pollack, M. M., Patel, K. M., & Ruttimann, U. E. (1996). PRISM III: An updated pediatric risk of mortality score. *Critical Care Medicine, 24*(5), 743–752. Retrieved from http://www.ncbi.nlm.nih.gov/pubmed/8706448

Pollack, M. M., Ruttimann, U. E., & Getson, P. R. (1988). Pediatric risk of mortality (PRISM) score. *Critical Care Medicine, 16*(11), 1110–1116.

Population and Demographics. (2016). Retrieved from https://www.rightplace.org/data-center/population-and-demographics

Randolph, A. G., Zollo, M. B., Wigton, R. S., & Yeh, T. S. (1997). Factors explaining variability among caregivers in the intent to restrict life-support interventions in a pediatric intensive care unit. *Critical Care Medicine, 25*(3), 435–439. Retrieved from http://www.ncbi.nlm.nih.gov/pubmed/9118659

Rees, G., Gledhill, J., Garralda, M. E., & Nadel, S. (2004). Psychiatric outcome following paediatric intensive care unit (PICU) admission: A cohort study. *Intensive Care Medicine, 30*(8), 1607–1614. https://doi.org/10.1007/s00134-004-2310-9

Reeves, E., Timmons, S., & Dampier, S. (2006). Parents' experiences of negotiating care for their technology-dependent child. *Journal of Child Health Care, 10*(3), 228–239. https://doi.org/10.1177/1367493506066483

Rosenman, M. B., Vik, T., Hui, S. L., & Breitfeld, P. P. (2005). Hospital resource utilization in childhood cancer. *Journal of Pediatric Hematology/Oncology, 27*(6), 295–300. Retrieved from http://www.ncbi.nlm.nih.gov/pubmed/15956880

Schneider, D. T., Lemburg, P., Sprock, I., Heying, R., Gobel, U., & Nurnberger, W. (2000). Introduction of the oncological pediatric risk of mortality score (O-PRISM) for ICU support following stem cell transplantation in children. *Bone Marrow Transplantation, 25*(10), 1079–1086. https://doi.org/10.1038/sj.bmt.1702403

Shudy, M., de Almeida, M. L., Ly, S., Landon, C., Groft, S., Jenkins, T. L., & Nicholson, C. E. (2006). Impact of pediatric critical illness and injury on families: A systematic literature review. *Pediatrics, 118*(Suppl 3), S203–S218. https://doi.org/10.1542/peds.2006-0951B

Siow, E., Wypij, D., Berry, P., Hickey, P., & Curley, M. A. (2013). The effect of continuity in nursing care on patient outcomes in the pediatric intensive care unit. *The Journal of Nursing Administration, 43*(7–8), 394–402. https://doi.org/10.1097/NNA.0b013e31829d61e5

Steliarova-Foucher, E., Stiller, C., Kaatsch, P., Berrino, F., Coebergh, J. W., Lacour, B., & Parkin, M. (2004). Geographical patterns and time trends of cancer incidence and survival among children and adolescents in Europe since the 1970s (the ACCISproject): An epidemiological study. *Lancet, 364*(9451), 2097–2105. https://doi.org/10.1016/S0140-6736(04)17550-8

Straehla, J. P., Barton, K. S., Yi-Frazier, J. P., Wharton, C., Baker, K. S., Bona, K., … Rosenberg, A. R. (2017). The benefits and burdens of cancer: A prospective longitudinal cohort study of adolescents and young adults. *Journal of Palliative Medicine*. https://doi.org/10.1089/jpm.2016.0369

Tukenova, M., Guibout, C., Oberlin, O., Doyon, F., Mousannif, A., Haddy, N., … de Vathaire, F. (2010). Role of cancer treatment in long-term overall and cardiovascular mortality after childhood cancer. *Journal of Clinical Oncology, 28*(8), 1308–1315. https://doi.org/10.1200/JCO.2008.20.2267

Wetzel, R. C., Sachedeva, R., & Rice, T. B. (2011). Are all ICUs the same? *Paediatric Anaesthesia, 21*(7), 787–793. https://doi.org/10.1111/j.1460-9592.2011.03595.x

Wiener, L., Hersh, S. P., & Alderfer, M. A. (2011). Psychiatric and psychosocial support for the child and family. In P. Pizzo & D. Poplack (Eds.), *Principles and practice of pediatric oncology* (6th ed., pp. 1323–1346). Philadelphia, PA: Lippincott Williams & Wilkins.

Zinter, M. S., DuBois, S. G., Spicer, A., Matthay, K., & Sapru, A. (2014). Pediatric cancer type predicts infection rate, need for critical care intervention, and mortality in the pediatric intensive care unit. *Intensive Care Medicine*, *40*(10), 1536–1544. https://doi.org/10.1007/s00134-014-3389-2

Chapter 8
The Impact of Childhood Cancer on the Quality of Life Among Healthy Siblings

Michelle Le and Tanya R. Fitzpatrick

Introduction

Cancer is the leading cause of death worldwide (WHO, 2017). For children aged 5–14 years, cancer is the second leading cause of death following accidents. In both Europe and the United States, incidence rates of childhood cancer have shown an increase over time since the middle of the last century (Steliarova-Foucher et al., 2004). However, in the United States, it was observed that death rates for all childhood and adolescent cancers combined have steadily declined by an average of 2.1% per year since 1975, resulting in an overall decline of more than 50% (Ward, DeSantis, Robbins, Kohler, & Jemal, 2014). Recent advancements in treatment have increased the overall 5-year survival rate for childhood cancers to approximately 80%.

The diagnosis of cancer in children and adolescents is a life altering event for many patients and their families. The most common cancers among children and adolescents vary by age. From a recent American Cancer Society study, the most common cancers in children aged 0–14 years are acute lymphoblastic leukemia (ALL), brain and central nervous system (CNS) tumors, neuroblastoma, and non-Hodgkin lymphoma (NHL). Hodgkin lymphoma (HL), thyroid carcinoma, brain and CNS tumors, and testicular germ cell tumors are the four most common cancers diagnosed in adolescents aged 15–19. The top three cancers among childhood survivors overall are ALL, brain and CNS tumors, and HL (Ward et al., 2014). Cancer incidence, mortality, and survival rates also vary by race and ethnicity. Non-Hispanic white (white) and Hispanic children have the highest incidence rates for childhood

M. Le (✉)
McGill University, Montreal, QC, Canada
e-mail: michelle.le@mail.mcgill.ca

T. R. Fitzpatrick
Department of Social work, Arizona State University, Westmount, QC, Canada

T. R. Fitzpatrick (ed.), *Quality of Life Among Cancer Survivors*,
https://doi.org/10.1007/978-3-319-75223-5_8

and adolescent cancers. Unlike many adult cancers, childhood and adolescent cancer incidence is not consistently higher among populations with lower socioeconomic status (Kroll, Stiller, Murphy, & Carpenter, 2011; Pan, Daniels, & Zhu, 2010). In general, the incidence of pediatric cancer is higher in industrialized countries than in developing countries, but international patterns differ by cancer type for reasons that are unknown (Bunin, 2004; Stiller & Parkin, 1996). While a considerable amount of research has been conducted on the quality of life among childhood cancer survivors and their family members in general, few studies have addressed the quality of life of siblings of cancer survivors (Carr-Gregg & White, 1987). Therefore, the purpose of this chapter is to examine the impact of childhood cancer on the quality of life (QOL) among healthy siblings.

In order to illustrate the impact of childhood cancer on QOL of healthy siblings, this chapter will be organized as follows:

1. Sample demographics
2. Literature review
3. Theories of sibling relationships
4. Therapeutic interventions
5. Implications

Sample Demographics

Due to the limited amount of research conducted regarding siblings of childhood cancer survivors, siblings under 18 years of age will come from various backgrounds of different races, religions, and living and economic arrangements. In this chapter, sibling criteria are not limited to age, gender, ethnicity, family structure, and types of childhood cancer diagnosis.

Literature Review

Health-Related Quality of Life

Health-related quality of life (HRQOL) is defined as a multidimensional construct covering physical, emotional, mental, social, and behavioral components of well-being (Davis et al., 2006). Numerous tools have been developed to assess quality of life for both pediatric and adult patient populations. For the pediatric population in particular, the PedsQL Measurement Model for Pediatric Quality of Life (Varni, Seid, & Rode, 1999) is a popular tool used in numerous research studies. The PedsQL was originally derived from data collected for a measurement and prediction study of HRQOL in children with cancer. Physical, emotional, social, and school functioning are all identified factors in the PedsQL Measurement Model that affect HRQOL among children. These factors represent the core dimensions of health as delineated by the World Health Organization. Physical functioning refers to the functional status in activities of daily living, while emotional functioning refers to the assessment of emotional distress. Interpersonal functioning in peer relations and in-school performance is assessed in social and school functioning, respectfully. Although the PedsQL was originally developed with cancer patients, the measured factors are applicable to a broad range of pediatric conditions and thus can be considered to study the HRQOL of healthy siblings of childhood cancer survivors.

Quality of Life Among Healthy Siblings

The impact of childhood cancer on the quality of life of healthy siblings continues to be an underreported area of concern. Knowledge about siblings is currently limited in amount, scope, and conclusiveness (Wilkins & Woodgate, 2005). Previous studies have shown that siblings have increased emotional distress, trouble with social interactions, and diminished in-school performance during the time of the childhood cancer diagnosis.

The diagnosis of cancer, with or without a cure, can have devastating effects on both the patients and their families (Bjork, Wiebe, & Hallstrom, 2005). When a child has cancer, healthcare providers often focus on helping the parent(s) and the sick child cope with the diagnosis and treatment (Deatrick et al., 2006; Giovanola, 2005). While the psychosocial care of these children has received increasing attention and emphasis in medical literature, the quality of life of siblings of such patients is an underreported area (Carr-Gregg & White, 1987). Previous studies have shown that the childhood cancer experience is a stressor that may increase subjective feelings of stress among healthy siblings and in some cases lead to decreased psychosocial competencies and increased psychopathology (J. S. Murray, 1999). Gaining insight and understanding the cancer experience, particularly from the perspective of siblings, can facilitate the development of knowledge that may be useful for oncologists, other healthcare professionals, and family members who provide care for siblings of children with cancer. Furthermore, knowledge about siblings' individual responses and perceptions of the cancer experience may also provide greater insight into the experiences of the family as a whole.

Theories of Sibling Relationships

Several psychological theories have been developed to explain multiple aspects of sibling relationships. Understanding the psychoanalytic-evolutionary perspective of sibling theories allows for further understanding of the impact of childhood cancer on the quality of life of healthy siblings. From a psychoanalytic-evolutionary perspective, John Bowlby's attachment theory (Bowlby, 1969) and Adler's theory of individual psychology (Ansbacher & Ansbacher, 1956) can be used to help explain the dynamics of sibling relationship.

Attachment Theory

Attachment theory was proposed by John Bowlby, in 1969, in an effort to explain the early bond between infants and their primary caregivers as critical to the infants' survival. Beginning in the first days of life, infants convey the need for their caregivers through their innate behavior, such as crying and clinging. Across their first year of life, an attachment relationship forms between infant and caregiver and varies in degree of security depending on the sensitivity and responsiveness of the infant's caregiver. In the second year of life, the attachment figure, the caregiver, may become a secure base from which children explore the world around them and return to in stressful circumstances for comfort and a sense of security. Separation or the loss of an attachment figure would give rise to a sense of anxiety and distress. Typically, the primary caregiver of the child is the mother, and she thus becomes the attachment figure. However, in addition to forming attachment relationships with their primary caregiver, children can form attachment relationships with a range of other common figures in their social environment. Siblings, for example, are common figures with which children may form attachment relationships given their presence in the child's everyday life. Early in life, the need for a sense of security means that attachment relationships are based on others' responsiveness to infants' needs, and thus sensitive and involved older siblings may become objects of attachment (Whiteman, McHale, & Soli, 2011). In addition to their primary caregivers, some children may use their brothers and sisters as a secure base from which to explore or as a source of comfort in stressful circumstances depending on the degree of sensitivity and responsiveness of the child's sibling. Consistent with the potential of siblings to serve as attachment figures, Jenkins (1992) found that some siblings turn to each other for emotional support in the face of parents' marital conflict (Jenkins, 1992). Other studies have also demonstrated the role of siblings as a source of emotional security at different points in life (Kim, McHale, Wayne Osgood, & Crouter, 2006).

Attachment theory may be used to explain the impact of childhood cancer on the HRQOL of healthy siblings. With the diagnosis of childhood cancer, family life is typically disrupted. Parents usually alter their activity levels and daily schedules in order to accommodate for the ill child's needs. As result, siblings tend to be overlooked and spend less time with their parents and more time with parental substitutes such as grandparents and neighbors (Barrera, 2000; Freeman, O'Dell, & Meola, 2000). From the attachment theory perspective, removal of attachment figures may result in a decline in emotional functioning as the key sources of emotional stability are removed from the sibling. Furthermore, the disruption of children's familial bonds with their primary caregivers and siblings may have long-term implications on the quality of their relationships where relationship insecurities may lead to conflictual, distant, or otherwise less satisfying relations.

Adler's Theory of Individual Psychology

Adler's (1924) theory of individual psychology aims to describe the process of sibling differentiation in relation to family dynamics. According to Adler, rivalry between siblings is grounded in each child's need to overcome potential feelings of inferiority. As a means of reducing competition, siblings often differentiate or deidentify as they develop different personal qualities and choose different niches. Parents recognize differences between their children in behavior, personality, and needs, and they often cite children's personal characteristics as motivation for treating their offspring differently (Crouter & Booth, 2003). According to Adler, parents' differential treatment of siblings and parental favoritism of one sibling over the other is linked to poorer sibling relationships. Adler's insights led him to advocate for the equal treatment of siblings as an important preventive measure in promoting self-esteem. A growing body of evidence is consistent with Adler's theory suggesting that parental differential treatment is linked to less positive sibling relationships from early childhood through adolescence (Brody, Stoneman, & Burke, 1987; Shanahan, McHale, Crouter, & Osgood, 2008; Stocker, Dunn, & Plomin, 1989). Also consistent with Adler's theory, previous studies have shown that sibling relationships were most positive when parents treated siblings equally (Boll, Ferring, & Filipp, 2003). Although more research needs to be conducted, implications of differential treatment remain an important avenue for future research. Equal treatment would seem like an important goal, but it can be very difficult to pursue due to the increasing time and demands placed on the parents to care for a seriously ill child with cancer.

Adler's theory of individual psychology has important implications in the long-term effects of childhood cancer as result of a sibling's HRQOL. Given the shift in parents' attention to the ill child needs after the cancer diagnosis, siblings are often overlooked and expected to adapt to the quick change in family dynamics. Siblings, however, may perceive this change in dynamics as parental favoritism of the child who is ill. Consistent with Adler's theory, siblings often experience feelings of rejection, anxiety, anger, jealousy, and animosity toward the ill sibling while dealing with the shift in parental attention (Wilkins & Woodgate, 2005). These feelings will ultimately be a key source of long-term sibling differentiation in family dynamics. As result, on a psychological and emotional level, the long-term impact of childhood cancer on the siblings' development may be explained by Adler's theory of individual psychology. For further illustration of this concept, please refer to a book by Jodi Picoult, 2005, entitled *My Sister's Keeper* which describes in detail the relationship a healthy sibling has with her parents and her older sister who is dying of cancer. Of the two theories, attachment theory (Bowlby, 1969) provides a pertinent, multifaceted explanation of siblings' HRQOL and is thus is an important theory in understanding the complex nature of sibling relationships and quality of life when another sibling in the family has cancer.

Health-Related Quality of Life

The measures of health-related quality of life (HRQOL) encompass physical functioning, emotional functioning, social functioning, and school functioning (Varni et al. (1999)). Physical functioning refers to the functional status of activities of daily living. Factors such as difficulty walking, running, doing sports, exercising, hurting, and having low energy are used to determine the functional status of activities of daily living. Emotional functioning assesses emotional distress where feelings of being afraid, sad, angry, and worried are indications of emotional distress. Functioning within interpersonal relationships is used to reflect social functioning. Having trouble getting along with other kids, not having any friends, being teased, and inability to keep up in child's play are among factors that determine functioning within interpersonal relationships. Finally, performance in school is evidently used to assess school functioning. Problems with paying attention in class, forgetting things, having trouble keeping up with homework, and missing school may indicate problems with school functioning. As shown through Bowlby's and Adler's theories, diagnosis of childhood cancer affects healthy sibling on multiple levels. It would therefore not be surprising that the quality of life of both siblings and cancer survivors are affected in similar manners, although the impact of childhood cancer goes far beyond one's quality of life.

Emotional Functioning

Emotional functioning in siblings has been extensively described in the literature. Frequently mentioned emotional reactions toward the diagnosis of childhood cancer include feelings of sadness, loneliness, isolation, anxiety, rejection, jealousy, frustration, and anger (Houtzager, Grootenhuis, & Last, 1999). These intense feelings would be especially poignant shortly after the diagnosis, when the sense of shock was greatest, and the family was under maximum stress (Chesler, Allswede, & Barbarin, 1992).

An overwhelming number of articles report siblings feeling very sad (Chesler et al., 1992; Sloper, 2000; Woodgate, 2000). The feeling of sadness among siblings usually stems from the worry that the sick child would die, miss their parents, and miss the life that their family used to have (Wilkins & Woodgate, 2005). Sadness also evolves from siblings feeling guilty that they were not able to do enough for their brother or sister, especially with death as the outcome (Chesler et al., 1992), or even after an ill sibling had been successfully treated; these feelings of sadness may continue to persist in siblings (Woodgate, 2000). It is clear that the diagnosis of childhood cancer goes further than the period of the illness itself and may have a long-term impact on the siblings of these patients.

Feelings of loneliness may arise when parents and other family members become preoccupied with the sick child, and siblings are left on the periphery of family life (Kramer, 1984). In fact, some studies also note that emotional needs of siblings are least adequately met of all family members (Spinetta & Spinetta, 1981). According to Bowlby's (1969) attachment theory; as the siblings' figures of attachment are taken away from them, it is not surprising that feelings of loneliness arise in these children. Siblings also have the tendency to internalize problems following the diagnosis of cancer, which further propagates self-isolation (Barbarin et al., 1995; Cohen, Friedrich, Jaworski, Copeland, & Pendergrass, 1994; Sahler et al., 1994). This may be due to siblings often believing that they are not as important as their brother or sister who has cancer, and many siblings perceive themselves to be alone and have no one to express their feelings to (Wilkins & Woodgate, 2005).

Siblings tend to feel anxious as they worry for their brother's or sister's health, their own health, and their families' security (Wilkins & Woodgate, 2005). As siblings are typically sheltered from their brother's or sister's illness, they would often feel anxious as sometimes less information is given regarding the diagnosis, and they may feel that there is little that they could do to help their sibling. For example, one sibling reported "I felt helpless because I did not fully understand what was going on...I thought everyone who had [the leukemia] died. I began to collect information, books, and pamphlets" (J. Murray, 1998). Additionally, anxiety pertaining to family favoritism and rejection may escalate while the sibling is adapting to new family routines (Chesler et al., 1992).

Rejection and jealousy stem from increased attention toward the sick child by parents, other family members, and friends (Bendor, 1990; Kramer, 1984; Sloper, 2000; Yin & Twinn, 2004). Low self-esteem and internalized hostility arise from siblings who often feel unloved and not as important as the sick child (Bendor, 1990). Another example from a sibling reported:

> I began to feel hatred for my sister. I often thought if I got sick, maybe I too would receive presents and sympathy. My sister stood bathed in the spotlight, and I'd been thrown into the corner. I resented her. I thought everyone was totally insensitive to me. People would always ask me how she was doing, never how I was doing. I was suffering just as much as she was—not physically, but emotionally. I became very tough on the outside, but I was dying on the inside. (J. Murray, 1998)

Feelings of rejection and jealousy are consistent with attachment theory (Bowlby, 1969) as parental and sibling relationships deteriorate once the figures of attachment are removed.

Finally, feelings of frustration and anger stem from the disruption of family life. Siblings resent inequitable treatment from their parents and changes in family routines that are necessary to accommodate the rigorous treatment regimen and its potential complications (Wilkins & Woodgate, 2005).

The plethora of intense emotions felt by siblings is best described by Bowlby's theory. As shown in the literature, the removal of attachment figures results in a decline in emotional functioning. The disruption of children's relationships with their parents and siblings may cause a decline in the quality of their relationship where the long-term effects may include conflictual, distant, or otherwise less satisfying future relationships.

Physical Functioning

Effects of childhood cancer on the physical functioning of siblings are relatively less well-studied in the literature. However, in a series of studies done by Houtzager et al. (Houtzager, Grootenhuis, Caron, & Last, 2004; Houtzager, Grootenhuis, Hoekstra-Weebers, Caron, & Last, 2003; Houtzager, Grootenhuis, Hoekstra-Weebers, & Last, 2005), physical quality of life and motor skills were evaluated at 1, 6, and 24 months after cancer diagnosis. Examples of physical problems evaluated in this study are headaches, stomach aches, nausea, vomiting, or other undefined problems. Examples of motor skills evaluated in this study include limitations in walking, running, or energy. Younger children (7–11-year-olds) demonstrated poorer physical quality of life and motor skills compared to norms 1 and 24 months after the cancer diagnosis. However, adolescent siblings (13–18-year-olds) showed no significant differences from the control group on measures of physical quality of life and motor skills at 1, 6, or 24 months post-diagnosis. Overall, in all age groups, physical complaints and problems with motor skills occurred relatively more often than in reference groups.

Physical functioning can also be viewed as psychosomatic and somatic problems reported by siblings' parents. In a study conducted by La¨hteenma¨ki et al. (2004) (Lahteenmaki, Sjoblom, Korhonen, & Salmi, 2004), parents of 33 siblings of childhood cancer patients and healthy controls completed *Conners' Parent Rating Scale* which measures signs of physical distress such as headaches, stomach aches, nausea, vomiting, loose bowel, aches and pains, and muscle tension were investigated. Authors of this study found that siblings below school age (≤7 years) tended to present more psychosomatic problems and somatic problems soon after the cancer diagnosis in comparison with the control group. However, these symptoms became less apparent during follow-up, although statistical significance was not reached. School-aged children (8–15-year-olds), by contrast, had marginally more psychomotor problems at 3 months and significantly more symptoms at 12 months post-diagnosis compared to the control group. There was no difference in somatic and psychosomatic symptoms for preschool siblings compared to controls at 3 or 12 months post-diagnosis.

Interestingly, in a study investigating the physical function and well-being of siblings' conducted by Zeltzer et al. (1997), the authors suggest that there may be discrepancies between parent and child assessments. Although siblings in this study were found to be moderately healthy, a trend of parental underreporting of sibling health measures was found when compared to siblings' reports. Healthcare utilization also appeared to be reduced for siblings of children with cancer. Parents of siblings were less likely to seek medical help for a variety of medical conditions, for which the parents of control children would bring their child to a doctor. Specifically, in the study, only one fourth of siblings' parents would seek medical help if their non-cancer-diagnosed child had bad stomach pains, while over half of the control parents would do so. Focus of care for families of children is often limited to the child with cancer. As indicated, siblings may be overlooked in the process. Additionally, findings from this study suggest that decline in health and physical functioning in siblings may be underreported. Primary research studies investigating the health and physical function of healthy siblings should consider obtaining responses from primary sources (i.e., the siblings when possible) supplemented with responses from secondary sources (i.e., the parents and other family members) in order to accurately obtain data.

In sum, the effect of childhood cancer on the physical functioning of siblings remains inconclusive. Further research on the physical functioning of siblings must be conducted to capture the full impact of childhood cancer on the health-related quality of life.

Social Functioning

Changes in siblings' social functioning may be expected after the diagnosis of childhood cancer. However, a recent study done by Alderfer et al. (2015) indicates that peer relationships of siblings of children with cancer are similar to their classmates (control group). Specifically, peer reports indicated no differences between siblings and other classmates in terms of social reputation, number of friendships, reciprocated friendships, or peer acceptance. Moreover, self-reported prosocial behavior and teacher-reported likability were higher for siblings in comparison with their peers. Self-reported loneliness, friendship quality, and perceived social support did not differ between the two groups. Several articles show findings similar to those of Alderfer et al. (2015). In multiple studies, there are no differences in the social functioning between siblings and control group based on parent, teacher, or self-reported measures (Buizer, de Sonneville, van den Heuvel-Eibrink, & Veerman, 2006; Dolgin et al., 1997; Lahteenmaki, Huostila, Hinkka, & Salmi, 2002; Packman et al., 1997; Packman et al., 2004; Packman et al., 2005; Zeltzer et al., 2008). Although the majority of articles find no significant social functioning deficits in siblings, some studies have indicated a decline in social functioning only in particular subgroups of siblings (Houtzager et al., 2003; Houtzager et al., 2004; Lahteenmaki et al., 2004). For instance, a study done by Houtzager et al. in 2003 demonstrated that of children aged 7–11 years, a substantial number of siblings report an impaired social quality of life compared to the reference group 2 years after the diagnosis of childhood cancer. Adolescent siblings aged 11–18, by contrast, showed no significant differences in terms of social quality of life compared to the reference group. The difference in results between children and adolescents may be due to adolescents' maturity and greater ability for social adaptation in the face of illness in the family. Few studies show siblings to have a poorer social functioning than their control group within a clinically significant range (Houtzager et al., 2005; Labay & Walco, 2004). Noted by many authors, even ones who found no differences in the social functioning of siblings and control groups, the decline in social functioning may be due to the decreased number of social opportunities when families change their routine in order to accommodate the ill child (Freeman et al., 2000; J. S. Murray, 2002; Sidhu, Passmore, & Baker, 2005; Sloper, 2000). Attachment theory can also explain the decline in social function in certain sibling subgroups. Disruption in the process of attachment to key figures, especially in younger children, may cause siblings to have difficulty getting along with others and be unable to develop a sense of confidence or trust in others. Children who are slow to adjust or are shy or irritable are likely to experience conflict with their parents and are less likely to receive parental acceptance or encouragement, which can make the children feel inadequate or unworthy (Hong & Park, 2012). Overall, social functioning of siblings is comparable to their peers. However, decline in social functioning of certain sibling subgroups is noted in several articles warrants further research.

School Functioning

Siblings' functioning in the school setting has also been investigated. One of the first primary research studies investigating this topic was conducted by Fife, Norton, & Groom (1987). In this study, increased absenteeism was reported for 6 of 31 siblings (19%), and a decline in academic performance was noticed for 17 of the siblings (55%) after the cancer diagnosis in comparison with the year prior to the diagnosis. In-school behavior problems such as withdrawal, deterioration in self-confidence, and anxiety were also observed in 17 siblings (55%). When examining the literature as a whole, two similar themes emerged in siblings with regard to school functioning: (1) disruptions in school performance and behavior and (2) the need to be more independent and responsible for own schoolwork. In regards to changes in school behavior, several studies have indicated that siblings experience more difficulties than the control group on measures of parent-reported and self-reported school functioning including concentration, memory, and learning (Houtzager et al., 2005; Labay & Walco, 2004; Lahteenmaki et al., 2004; Packman et al., 2004; Packman et al., 2005). These disruptions in school performance and behavior may be due to changes in routine, fatigue, worry, lack of parental support, and lack of help with schoolwork. Although most studies show a negative change in school performance and behavior, other studies report conflicting results showing no differences in rates of repeating school grades, teacher-reported school performance, attention and learning problems, study skills, parent-reported attention problems or self-reported concentration, and memory and learning problems. Studies showing no differences in school performance or behavior usually consist of samples who are farther away from date of childhood cancer diagnosis in comparison with studies that show negative changes in school performance and behavior (Buizer et al., 2006; Houtzager et al., 2004; Manne & Miller, 1998; Mulrooney et al., 2008; Packman et al., 1997). Overall, numerous studies have indicated that problems in school performance or behavior typically arise 1–24 months post-diagnosis (Houtzager et al., 2005; Labay & Walco, 2004; Lahteenmaki et al., 2004). Notably, in two studies, the siblings of pediatric cancer patients showed more distress in their school functioning than the patients themselves (Cairns, Clark, Smith, & Lansky, 1979; Fife, Norton, & Groom, 1987).

Summary of Literature Review

Overall, the impact of childhood cancer on a healthy siblings' HRQOL is extremely complex with a number of short- and long-term consequences. John Bowlby's (1969) theory of attachment provides a useful theory to explain the studies that were reviewed in this chapter. With the diagnosis of childhood cancer in the family, the healthy siblings' emotional range is sometimes restricted to sadness, loneliness, isolation, anxiety, rejection, jealousy, frustration, and anger. The effect of childhood cancer on the physical functioning of healthy siblings remains inconclusive and warrants further research. A decline in social functioning in certain sibling subgroups, particularly in younger siblings, was also noted. Problems in school performance or behavior typically arise 1–24 months post-diagnosis. The diagnosis of childhood cancer impacts all four spheres of a healthy siblings' HRQOL. Given the potentially harmful implications of these results, further research on siblings of childhood cancer survivors is warranted.

Therapeutic Interventions

Familial routines and interactions will differ when a child is diagnosed with cancer. Said changes can be especially challenging and stressful for the sick child's healthy siblings. Yet, at times, a cancerous child can have a positive effect on a healthy sibling. The child who is well may portray more signs of compassion, positivity, generosity, and/or being helpful (Alderfer et al., 2015). While there is the possibility that a terribly ill child can positively impact a healthy sibling, often, the healthy sibling will yield negative effects. These negative effects can result in the sibling feeling depressed, withdrawn, anxious, fearful, angry, and isolated (Houtzager et al., 1999). Coping with the stressors brought on by a child's cancer diagnosis is crucial to the maintenance of well-being. A few coping mechanisms including communication, social support and recognition of sibling's health, counseling, maintaining hobbies, and keeping consistent routines have been proven to be effective in reducing and making the negative emotions less severe in healthy siblings.

Communication

Communication among family members is key to aiding the family adjust to the necessary attention an illness like cancer demands. Lower levels of communication hold the typical outcome of the healthy sibling experiencing misunderstandings and the potential to have all negative feelings mentioned previously. Conversely, higher levels of communication between healthy siblings and their parents have been shown to have a positive relationship (Breyer, Kunin, Kalish, & Patenaude, 1993; Havermans & Eiser, 1994). Thus, open and honest discussions are crucial to protect healthy siblings from the suffering of destructive thoughts, feelings, and emotions. Families that have grown closer in the face of illness have been successful in doing so as they have empathized and learned to support one another (Chesler et al., 1992; Kramer, 1984). It is very important to understand that each person has a different way of coping with the way in which they feel. The more parents understand the way the sibling expresses themselves, the more they can aid in said child's coping. Thus, oncology and healthcare providers may aid and promote more open communication between family members, siblings, and children with cancer by participating in family support groups and family team meetings.

Social Support and Ventilation of Feelings

Parents have been found to play an incredibly important role in a healthy sibling's support system. Siblings tend to resort to emotional expression when dealing with how they feel. An un-ill child may have difficulty in initiating conversations with their parents as the feeling of guilt frequently occurs. Siblings may feel guilty for wanting attention and having their emotions validated and their needs met (Chesler et al., 1992). Demonstrating support by listening, empathizing, and allowing the healthier child to vent about their thoughts and emotions will allow all to better understand the sibling's otherwise repressed feelings of negativity (Alderfer et al., 2015). Children with cancer are not the only ones who are hurting, their healthy siblings suffer as well. Spending time simply talking with the sibling can yield positive results including strengthening their social skills, improve familial bonding, and decrease emotional instability.

Counseling

Having a child ill with cancer can be an incredibly heavy burden for siblings and all family members. Despite one's best efforts to maintain familial balance, a healthy sibling may require extra support from a counselor such as a mental health specialist, psychiatrist, oncology social worker, or a psychologist. As a trained professional, counselors can provide therapy through talking about one's overwhelming situation. Counseling can help healthy siblings, parents, and families alike to manage the many challenges brought on by having a child with cancer (Last & Grootenhuis, 1998). The environment provided by a counselor generally promotes one's confidence in voicing up concerns and troubling feelings and allows siblings to feel safe in one's own self-expression (NIH, 2013). This helps healthy siblings of cancer-diagnosed children to focus on positively managing and adjusting to their new life dynamics as opposed to suffering in negative feelings.

Hobbies

To stay physically fit is very important for one's health. Healthy siblings may not be as healthy after giving so much attention to the sickly child. With all added emotional stressors, the sibling can easily forget to take care of themselves (Houtzager et al., 1999). The healthy sibling should continue to take part in extracurricular activities they enjoyed prior to the diagnosis. Without a hobby to enjoy, life can become incredibly demanding and draining upon one's emotional and mental health. Pursing a hobby can have numerous benefits such as relaxation, allowing one to network, and can help one stay physically active (NIH, 2013). Having the healthy sibling pursue a hobby, such as a sport or an art, that they enjoy allows them to solely focus on a task they love for a certain time. During this allocated time, it is necessary for the sibling to concentrate on the task at hand and thus will not allow them to be distracted by negative thoughts and other issues occurring in their lives. Hobbies, especially those done in teams, force one to have social interactions and communicate with others. This can have a great positive impact on the healthy sibling's social life, ensuring one is not isolated and feeling abandoned. A hobby that doubles as a sport can be physically rewarding in terms of body weight and shape, as well as it can be enjoyable. Achieving goals within the sibling's choice of activity can increase self-esteem and self-confidence. Having higher self-esteem and confidence leads away from depression, anxiety, and other mental health illnesses (NIH, 2013).

Keeping Consistent Routines

The maintenance of consistency is important in any child's life, and it is even more so in that of a sibling to a child with cancer. Having an established routine will be a reliever of stress and can aid the sibling to more easily adapt to changed family dynamics (NIH, 2013). Established schedules provide a sense of security for siblings by having consistency in expectations. This also allows them to develop the skill of self-discipline despite the parents'/caregivers' potential unavailability. Furthermore, having scheduled family time is helpful as it allows siblings to spend quality time with their parents, as well as continuing the development of their relationships even with an altered family dynamic.

Implications for Healthcare Providers

Siblings are often overlooked in the presence of an ill child. Especially for healthcare providers in the oncology field, it is easy to forget the effect of childhood cancer on other members of the family when they may not overtly show signs or symptoms of distress. Recognizing that the HRQOL of siblings is negatively affected in the face of cancer is the first step toward providing holistic care for the ill patients and their sibling counterparts. Being aware of community social services available for the siblings is the next step. Pediatric social workers are typically well-equipped to follow siblings and their families during a time of shifting family dynamics. Further, social workers are well aware of community services and activities that siblings can benefit from. Multidisciplinary pediatric centers are also a great resource for at-risk siblings to be referred to during vulnerable periods. These pediatric centers typically work in a milieu where physicians, social support workers, and psychologists collaborate to provide quality of care for the child. As social services for siblings typically vary by community, it is encouraged that healthcare professionals are kept up to date with community resources.

Discussion

The literature review in this chapter provides a number of important insights on the impact of childhood cancer on the HRQOL of healthy siblings. The attachment theory by Bowlby (1969) attempts to explain some of the findings from the literature studies for sibling HRQOL. The studies from this chapter demonstrate that childhood cancer can negatively affect all four spheres, emotional, physical, social, and school functioning, of HRQOL in healthy siblings. Our findings reveal that childhood cancer plays a crucial role in the short-term HRQOL, while there are indications that it may have an important role in the long-term HRQOL of non-ill siblings. Multiple therapeutic interventions such as communication, social support and ventilation of feelings, counseling, hobbies, and keeping consistent routines have been proven to help siblings cope with the change in familial routines, post-diagnosis. Although this research is promising, said research is still in its infancy, and more studies are required to fully understand the impact of childhood cancer on healthy siblings as a whole.

Acknowledgments The authors would like to thank Clara Le for her help with the Therapeutic Interventions section.

References

Adler, A. (1924). Alfred Asler's theory of individual psychology. In: A. Adler (ed), Wikipedia. ISBN: 9781136330094.

Alderfer, M. A., Stanley, C., Conroy, R., Long, K. A., Fairclough, D. L., Kazak, A. E., & Noll, R. B. (2015). The social functioning of siblings of children with cancer: A multi-informant investigation. *Journal of Pediatric Psychology, 40*(3), 309–319. https://doi.org/10.1093/jpepsy/jsu079

Ansbacher, H. L., & Ansbacher, R. R. (1956). The individual psychology of Alfred Adler. Oxford, England: BasicBooks Inc.

Barbarin, O. A., Sargent, J. R., Sahler, O. J. Z., Carpenter, P. J., Copeland, D. R., Dolgin, M. J., ... Zeltzer, L. (1995). Sibling adaptation to childhood cancer collaborative study. *Journal of Psychosocial Oncology, 13*(3), 1–20. https://doi.org/10.1300/J077V13N03_01

Barrera, M. (2000). Brief clinical report: Procedural pain and anxiety management with mother and sibling as co-therapists. *Journal of Pediatric Psychology, 25*(2), 117–121.

Bendor, S. J. (1990). Anxiety and isolation in siblings of pediatric cancer patients: The need for prevention. *Social Work in Health Care, 14*(3), 17–35. https://doi.org/10.1300/J010v14n03_02

Bjork, M., Wiebe, T., & Hallstrom, I. (2005). Striving to survive: families' lived experiences when a child is diagnosed with cancer. *Journal of Pediatric Oncology Nursing, 22*(5), 265–275. https://doi.org/10.1177/1043454205279303

Boll, T., Ferring, D., & Filipp, S. H. (2003). Perceived parental differential treatment in middle adulthood: Curvilinear relations with individuals' experienced relationship quality to sibling and parents. *Journal of Family Psychology, 17*(4), 472–487. https://doi.org/10.1037/0893-3200.17.4.472

Bowlby, J. (1969). Attachment and loss v. 3 (Vol. 1). Random House. Furman, W., & Buhrmester, D. (2009). *Methods and measures: The network of relationships inventory: Behavioral systems version. International Journal of Behavioral Development, 33*, 470–478.

Breyer, J., Kunin, H., Kalish, L. A., & Patenaude, A. F. (1993). The adjustment of siblings of pediatric cancer patients—A sibling and parent perspective. *Psychooncology, 2*(3), 201–208. https://doi.org/10.1002/pon.2960020306

Brody, G. H., Stoneman, Z., & Burke, M. (1987). Child temperaments, maternal differential behavior, and sibling relationships. *Developmental Psychology, 23*(3), 354.

Buizer, A. I., de Sonneville, L. M., van den Heuvel-Eibrink, M. M., & Veerman, A. J. (2006). Behavioral and educational limitations after chemotherapy for childhood acute lymphoblastic leukemia or Wilms tumor. *Cancer, 106*(9), 2067–2075. https://doi.org/10.1002/cncr.21820

Bunin, G. R. (2004). Nongenetic causes of childhood cancers: Evidence from international variation, time trends, and risk factor studies. *Toxicology and Applied Pharmacology, 199*(2), 91–103. https://doi.org/10.1016/j.taap.2003.12.028

Cairns, N. U., Clark, G. M., Smith, S. D., & Lansky, S. B. (1979). Adaptation of siblings to childhood malignancy. *The Journal of Pediatrics, 95*(3), 484–487.

Carr-Gregg, M., & White, L. (1987). Siblings of paediatric cancer patients: A population at risk. *Medical and Pediatric Oncology, 15*(2), 62–68.

Chesler, M. A., Allswede, J., & Barbarin, O. O. (1992). Voices from the margin of the family. *Journal of Psychosocial Oncology, 9*(4), 19–42. https://doi.org/10.1300/J077v09n04_02

Cohen, D. S., Friedrich, W. N., Jaworski, T. M., Copeland, D., & Pendergrass, T. (1994). Pediatric cancer: Predicting sibling adjustment. *Journal of Clinical Psychology, 50*(3), 303–319.

Crouter, A. C., & Booth, A. (2003). *Children's influence on family dynamics: The neglected side of family relationships*. Mahwah, NJ: Routledge.

Davis, E., Waters, E., Mackinnon, A., Reddihough, D., Graham, H. K., Mehmet-Radji, O., & Boyd, R. (2006). Paediatric quality of life instruments: A review of the impact of the conceptual framework on outcomes. *Developmental Medicine and Child Neurology, 48*(4), 311–318. https://doi.org/10.1017/s0012162206000673

Deatrick, J. A., Thibodeaux, A. G., Mooney, K., Schmus, C., Pollack, R., & Davey, B. H. (2006). Family management style framework: A new tool with potential to assess families who have children with brain tumors. *Journal of Pediatric Oncology Nursing*, *23*(1), 19–27.

Dolgin, M. J., Blumensohn, R., Mulhern, R. K., Orbach, J., Sahler, O. J., Roghmann, K. J., … Copeland, D. R. (1997). Sibling adaptation to childhood cancer collaborative study. *Journal of Psychosocial Oncology*, *15*(1), 1–14. https://doi.org/10.1300/J077v15n01_01

Fife, B., Norton, J., & Groom, G. (1987). The family's adaptation to childhood leukemia. *Social Science & Medicine*, *24*(2), 159–168. https://doi.org/10.1016/0277-9536(87)90248-6

Freeman, K., O'Dell, C., & Meola, C. (2000). Issues in families of children with brain tumors. *Oncology Nursing Forum*, *27*(5), 843–848.

Giovanola, J. (2005). Sibling involvement at the end of life. *Journal of Pediatric Oncology Nursing*, *22*(4), 222–226. https://doi.org/10.1177/1043454205276956

Havermans, T., & Eiser, C. (1994). Siblings of a child with cancer. *Child: Care, Health and Development*, *20*(5), 309–322.

Hong, Y. R., & Park, J. S. (2012). Impact of attachment, temperament and parenting on human development. *Korean Journal of Pediatrics*, *55*(12), 449–454. https://doi.org/10.3345/kjp.2012.55.12.449

Houtzager, B. A., Grootenhuis, M. A., Caron, H. N., & Last, B. F. (2004). Quality of life and psychological adaptation in siblings of paediatric cancer patients, 2 years after diagnosis. *Psychooncology*, *13*(8), 499–511. https://doi.org/10.1002/pon.759

Houtzager, B. A., Grootenhuis, M. A., Hoekstra-Weebers, J. E., Caron, H. N., & Last, B. F. (2003). Psychosocial functioning in siblings of paediatric cancer patients one to six months after diagnosis. *European Journal of Cancer*, *39*(10), 1423–1432.

Houtzager, B. A., Grootenhuis, M. A., Hoekstra-Weebers, J. E., & Last, B. F. (2005). One month after diagnosis: Quality of life, coping and previous functioning in siblings of children with cancer. *Child: Care, Health and Development*, *31*(1), 75–87. https://doi.org/10.1111/j.1365-2214.2005.00459.x

Houtzager, B. A., Grootenhuis, M. A., & Last, B. F. (1999). Adjustment of siblings to childhood cancer: A literature review. *Support Care Cancer*, *7*(5), 302–320.

Jenkins, J. (1992). *Sibling relationships in disharmonious homes: Potential difficulties and protective effects*. In F. Boer & J. Dunn (Eds.), Children's sibling relationships: Developmental and clinical issues (pp. 125–138). Hillsdale, US: Lawrence Erlbaum Associates, Inc.

Kim, J.-Y., McHale, S. M., Wayne Osgood, D., & Crouter, A. C. (2006). Longitudinal course and family correlates of sibling relationships from childhood through adolescence. *Child Development*, *77*(6), 1746–1761. https://doi.org/10.1111/j.1467-8624.2006.00971.x

Kramer, R. F. (1984). Living with childhood cancer: Impact on the healthy siblings. *Oncology Nursing Forum*, *11*(1), 44–51.

Kroll, M. E., Stiller, C. A., Murphy, M. F., & Carpenter, L. M. (2011). Childhood leukemia and socioeconomic status in England and Wales 1976-2005: Evidence of higher incidence in relatively affluent communities persists over time. *British Journal of Cancer*, *105*(11), 1783–1787. https://doi.org/10.1038/bjc.2011.415

Labay, L. E., & Walco, G. A. (2004). Brief report: Empathy and psychological adjustment in siblings of children with cancer. *Journal of Pediatric Psychology*, *29*(4), 309–314.

Lahteenmaki, P. M., Huostila, J., Hinkka, S., & Salmi, T. T. (2002). Childhood cancer patients at school. *European Journal of Cancer*, *38*(9), 1227–1240.

Lahteenmaki, P. M., Sjoblom, J., Korhonen, T., & Salmi, T. T. (2004). The siblings of childhood cancer patients need early support: A follow up study over the first year. *Archives of Disease in Childhood*, *89*(11), 1008–1013. https://doi.org/10.1136/adc.2002.012088

Last, B. F., & Grootenhuis, M. A. (1998). Emotions, coping and the need for support in families of children with cancer: A model for psychosocial care. *Patient Education and Counseling*, *33*(2), 169–179.

Manne, S., & Miller, D. (1998). Social support, social conflict, and adjustment among adolescents with cancer. *Journal of Pediatric Psychology*, *23*(2), 121–130.

Mulrooney, D. A., Dover, D. C., Li, S., Yasui, Y., Ness, K. K., Mertens, A. C., … Davies, S. M. (2008). Twenty years of follow-up among survivors of childhood and young adult acute myeloid leukemia: A report from the Childhood Cancer Survivor Study. *Cancer, 112*(9), 2071–2079. https://doi.org/10.1002/cncr.23405

Murray, J. (1998). The lived experience of childhood cancer: One sibling's perspective. *Issues in Comprehensive Pediatric Nursing, 21*(4), 217–227. https://doi.org/10.1080/014608698265429

Murray, J. S. (1999). Siblings of children with cancer: A review of the literature. *Journal of Pediatric Oncology Nursing, 16*(1), 25–34.

Murray, J. S. (2002). A qualitative exploration of psychosocial support for siblings of children with cancer. *Journal of Pediatric Nursing, 17*(5), 327–337.

National Cancer Institute, National Institutes of Health. (2013). When your brother or sister has cancer: A guide for teens. USA: CreateSpace Independent Publishing Platform.

Packman, W., Fine, J., Chesterman, B., vanZutphen, K., Golan, R., & Amylon, M. (2004). Camp Okizu: Preliminary investigation of a psychological intervention for siblings of pediatric cancer patients. *Children's Health Care, 33*(3), 201–215. https://doi.org/10.1207/s15326888chc3303_3

Packman, W., Greenhalgh, J., Chesterman, B., Shaffer, T., Fine, J., Van Zutphen, K., … Amylon, M. D. (2005). Siblings of pediatric cancer patients: The quantitative and qualitative nature of quality of life. *Journal of Psychosocial Oncology, 23*(1), 87–108. https://doi.org/10.1300/J077v23n01_06

Packman, W. L., Crittenden, M. R., Schaeffer, E., Bongar, B., Fischer, J. B., & Cowan, M. J. (1997). Psychosocial consequences of bone marrow transplantation in donor and nondonor siblings. *Journal of Developmental and Behavioral Pediatrics, 18*(4), 244–253.

Pan, I. J., Daniels, J. L., & Zhu, K. (2010). Poverty and childhood cancer incidence in the United States. *Cancer Causes & Control, 21*(7), 1139–1145. https://doi.org/10.1007/s10552-010-9528-3

Picoult, J. (2005). My sister's keeper: a novel. New York: Washington Square Press.

Sahler, O. J., Roghmann, K. J., Carpenter, P. J., Mulhern, R. K., Dolgin, M. J., Sargent, J. R., … Zeltzer, L. K. (1994). Sibling adaptation to childhood cancer collaborative study: Prevalence of sibling distress and definition of adaptation levels. *Journal of Developmental and Behavioral Pediatrics, 15*(5), 353–366.

Shanahan, L., McHale, S. M., Crouter, A. C., & Osgood, D. W. (2008). Linkages between parents' differential treatment, youth depressive symptoms, and sibling relationships. *Journal of Marriage and Family, 70*(2), 480–494.

Sidhu, R., Passmore, A., & Baker, D. (2005). An investigation into parent perceptions of the needs of siblings of children with cancer. *Journal of Pediatric Oncology Nursing, 22*(5), 276–287. https://doi.org/10.1177/1043454205278480

Sloper, P. (2000). Experiences and support needs of siblings of children with cancer. *Health & Social Care in the Community, 8*(5), 298–306. https://doi.org/10.1046/j.1365-2524.2000.00254.x

Spinetta, J., & Spinetta, P. (1981). *Living with childhood cancer*. St. Louis, MO: The C.V. Mosby.

Steliarova-Foucher, E., Stiller, C., Kaatsch, P., Berrino, F., Coebergh, J. W., Lacour, B., … Parkin, M. (2004). Geographical patterns and time trends of cancer incidence and survival among children and adolescents in Europe since the 1970s (the ACCIS project): An epidemiological study. *Lancet, 364*(9451), 2097–2105. https://doi.org/10.1016/s0140-6736(04)17550-8

Stiller, C. A., & Parkin, D. M. (1996). Geographic and ethnic variations in the incidence of childhood cancer. *British Medical Bulletin, 52*(4), 682–703.

Stocker, C., Dunn, J., & Plomin, R. (1989). Sibling relationships: Links with child temperament, maternal behavior, and family structure. *Child Development, 60*, 715–727.

Varni, J. W., Seid, M., & Rode, C. A. (1999). The PedsQL: Measurement model for the pediatric quality of life inventory. *Medical Care, 37*(2), 126–139.

Ward, E., DeSantis, C., Robbins, A., Kohler, B., & Jemal, A. (2014). Childhood and adolescent cancer statistics, 2014. *CA: A Cancer Journal for Clinicians, 64*(2), 83–103. https://doi.org/10.3322/caac.21219

Whiteman, S. D., McHale, S. M., & Soli, A. (2011). Theoretical perspectives on sibling relationships. *Journal of Family Theory & Review*, *3*(2), 124–139. https://doi.org/10.1111/j.1756-2589.2011.00087.x

WHO. (2017). Cancer Fact Sheet. Lyon, France: World Health Organization.

Wilkins, K. L., & Woodgate, R. L. (2005). A review of qualitative research on the childhood cancer experience from the perspective of siblings: A need to give them a voice. *Journal of Pediatric Oncology Nursing*, *22*(6), 305–319. https://doi.org/10.1177/1043454205278035

Woodgate, R. (2000). Part II: A critical review of qualitative research related to children's experiences with cancer. *Journal of Pediatric Oncology Nursing*, *17*(4), 207–228. https://doi.org/10.1177/104345420001700403

Yin, L. K., & Twinn, S. (2004). The effect of childhood cancer on Hong Kong Chinese families at different stages of the disease. *Cancer Nursing*, *27*(1), 17–24.

Zeltzer, L. K., Chen, E., Weiss, R., Guo, M. D., Robison, L. L., Meadows, A. T., … Byrne, J. (1997). Comparison of psychologic outcome in adult survivors of childhood acute lymphoblastic leukemia versus sibling controls: A cooperative Children's Cancer Group and National Institutes of Health study. *Journal of Clinical Oncology*, *15*(2), 547–556. https://doi.org/10.1200/jco.1997.15.2.547

Zeltzer, L. K., Lu, Q., Leisenring, W., Tsao, J. C., Recklitis, C., Armstrong, G., … Ness, K. K. (2008). Psychosocial outcomes and health-related quality of life in adult childhood cancer survivors: A report from the childhood cancer survivor study. *Cancer Epidemiology, Biomarkers & Prevention*, *17*(2), 435–446. https://doi.org/10.1158/1055-9965.epi-07-2541

Chapter 9
The Effect of Physical Activity on Post-Traumatic Stress Disorder Among Parents of Pediatric Cancer Survivors

Veronique Huot and Tanya R. Fitzpatrick

Introduction

As parents, having a child with a life-threatening illness can cause intense reactions (Landolt, Vollrath, Ribi, Gnehm, & Sennhauser, 2003). Evidence has shown that the journey through cancer can be extremely traumatic for the children and their parents (Kazak, Boeving, Alderfer, Hwang, & Reilly, 2005). Mothers and fathers of children with newly diagnosed cancer showed the highest rates of post-traumatic stress disorder (PTSD) compared with parents of children that have been diagnosed with diabetes (chronic illness) or with physical injuries (Landolt et al., 2003). PTSD is defined by the Canadian Mental Health Association as an illness that is often associated with a traumatic event that involves death or the threat of death. Individuals may show a variety of symptoms including mood swings, irritability, nervousness, flashbacks, insomnias, disconnection to reality, and much more. Furthermore, evidence suggests that PTSD is associated with cardiovascular disease, metabolic syndrome, obesity, and diabetes (Hall, Hoerster, & Yancy Jr, 2015; Rosenbaum et al., 2015). Other potential adverse consequences of PTSD mentioned in the literature include impaired psychological functioning, increased risk of suicide, and substance abuse among adults with current PTSD or sub-threshold diagnosis of primary PTSD (Rosenbaum, Vancampfort, et al., 2015).

According to a study, distress can be reduced by participation in physical activities among cancer survivors (Leimanis & Fitzpatrick, 2014). The purpose of this chapter is to explore via a literature review the relationship between physical activity and PTSD symptoms among parents of pediatric cancer patients. Physical activity

V. Huot (✉)
McGill University, Montreal, QC, Canada

T. R. Fitzpatrick
Department of Social Work, Arizona State University, Westmount, QC, Canada

T. R. Fitzpatrick (ed.), *Quality of Life Among Cancer Survivors*,
https://doi.org/10.1007/978-3-319-75223-5_9

is defined as any bodily movement produced by skeletal muscles in energy expenditure (Caspersen, Powell, & Christenson, 1985). It is important to examine physical activity as an intervention among parents of childhood cancer survivors. Previous studies have demonstrated that physical activity can have a large and beneficial effect on mental health (Hall et al., 2015) and has proven to decrease anxiety in humans (Asmundson et al., 2013). Physical activity has also been shown to have a relationship to PTSD (Powers et al., 2015). Exploring the impact of physical activity on PTSD symptoms in parents of pediatric cancer survivors provides further insight and knowledge for health-care professionals to promote physical activity in community or cancer support programs especially for the high-risk population of parents with children affected by cancer. The help provided to the primary caregiver of the child will directly help to inform better care and support for the pediatric patient.

The aims of the chapter will be addressed by focusing on the following:

- Post-traumatic stress disorder
- Theoretical perspectives, followed by literature on:
  (a) Childhood cancer
  (b) Parents of pediatric oncology patients
  (c) Physical activity
  (d) Physical activity and PTSD
  (e) Summary of the review
- Discussion:
  (a) Limitations
  (b) Implications for clinical practice
  (c) Future research

Post-Traumatic Stress Disorder (PTSD)

PTSD is a disorder caused by the exposure to a traumatic event resulting in the development of characteristic symptoms. It was previously classified under the "anxiety disorder" but is now, in the latest version of the *Diagnostic and Statistical Manual of Mental Disorder* (DSM-V), classified under "trauma and stress-related disorder." The diagnosis for a population over 6 years old is made out of height criteria (American.Psychiatric.Association, 2013). First, the individual must be exposed directly or indirectly (witness or close relative) to a traumatic event including (but not exclusively) actual or threatened to death, serious injury, or sexual violence. Second, the individual must be re-experiencing symptoms of the traumatic event such as recurrent, involuntary, and distressing memories or dreams or intense and distressing reactions of reminders of the trauma. Third, the individual persistently avoids or tries to avoid memories, feelings, places, persons, situations, objects, or anything else that could be a reminder of the traumatic event. Fourth, the individual will present with negative cognitive alterations as in amnesia, negative beliefs of oneself, negative emotional state, distortion of causes and consequences of the event, or diminished interest in others and less interest in participating in activities. Fifth, the individual will start being more reckless, irritable, hyper-vigilant, unable to focus, and sleep disturbed or have an exaggerated startle response. Sixth, the duration of all the symptoms usually lasts more than a month. Seventh, the distress will significantly impair the social, occupational, and functional part of the individual's life. Eight, the disturbance of the individual is not associated with any medical condition or any physiological effect (APA, 2013).

The prevalence of PTSD in the world ranges from 1.3% to 37.4% (Van Ameringen, Mancini, Patterson, & Boyle, 2008). The data found on Statistics Canada website is taken from the American Psychiatric Association's DSM-IV manual and other American sources. It reports a lifetime prevalence of PTSD of approximately 8% in the general population. According to a recent study conducted in Canada, the rate of lifetime PTSD was found to be 9.2%, and the current rate was 2.4% (Van Ameringen et al., 2008). Other findings from the same study reveal a tendency of higher prevalence rate in women (12.8%) than men (5%) in lifetime prevalence of PTSD. The majority of the participants also reported having post-traumatic symptoms that lasted more than a year (68.5%) (Van Ameringen et al., 2008).

PTSD has damaging consequences on the physical health, as well as the mental health of the parents (Asmundson et al., 2013; Fetzner & Asmundson, 2015; Hall et al., 2015; Rosenbaum, Vancampfort, et al., 2015). Additionally, PTSD is a prevalent and costly psychiatric disorder associated with high rates of obesity and cardiovascular and metabolic diseases (Hall et al., 2015). Anxiety disorders like PTSD also exert substantial economic strain on society (Asmundson et al., 2013) and a considerable high level of medical utilization (APA, 2013). DSM-V manual (APA, 2013) also reveals that PTSD is associated with emotional impairment and associated with suicide ideation and suicide attempts. In general, individuals with PTSD exhibit disturbance in social relationships and in day-to-day functioning (APA, 2013).

Further research on PTSD in Canada demonstrated that PTSD symptoms are often chronic (68.5% of the individuals in this study reported symptoms lasting more than a year) and associated with significant impairment and high rates of comorbidity which includes alcohol and/or drug abuse or dependence problems (Van Ameringen et al., 2008).

Theoretical Perspectives

Several theories were found to be applicable to help conceptualize and clarify the experience of childhood cancer as it relates to PTSD. This review tries to explore the current findings of cancer-related PTSD and PTSS in childhood cancer survivors and their parents and its relationship with physical activity. Post-traumatic stress symptoms (PTSS) are defined as specific symptoms that allow measurement of post-traumatic stress reactions and risk of PTSD diagnosis (Bruce, 2006). Two theories will be described: the activity theory and the pediatric model of traumatic stress (PMTS).

The *activity theory* proposes that a positive relationship exists between activity and life satisfaction and well-being (Maddox, 2001). The activity theory is built around four major concepts such as activity, equilibrium, adaptation to role loss, and life satisfaction (Maddox, 2001). Although Maddox developed the activity theory around the process of aging, the theory is also applicable to cancer. Cancer is an illness that completely and dramatically changes the life of the people affected by it. Equilibrium may be lost in the life of the parents. Suddenly, their whole life becomes focused on dealing with this illness and taking care of their child (Rabineau, Mabe, & Vega, 2008). Parents will often miss work to accompany their child for treatments. They will spend countless hours at the hospital by their child's bedside, and it is usually necessary to limit their daily life activities. A study in Sweden demonstrated that parents felt restricted in their everyday activities and forced to miss work or school a considerable amount of time. The percentage of restriction felt was ranging from 77 to 84% in the first 4 months after diagnosis (Hoven, Gronqvist, Poder, von Essen, & Lindahl Norberg, 2017). It was also suggested that parents who felt the higher level of restriction also had higher prevalence of PTSD. There is a need for role adaptation. Parents of a child with cancer are caregivers, but they are also workers, friends, and/or lovers. A person usually carries more than one role in their life, and when they have a child who is diagnosed with cancer, the role of caregiver takes over the other roles. Parents will often end up withdrawing from their community and society engagements to allow more time for their ill child. The activity theory supports a review conducted by Asmundson et al. (2013) which proposes that there is a positive benefit of breaking the isolation from society to include regular physical activity in one's day-to-day routine as a way to increase social interactions and increase life satisfaction (Asmundson et al., 2013; Maddox, 2001).

PTSD usually happens with traumatic events that disrupt ones equilibrium and state of well-being. The concept of the activity theory helps to clarify the possible association between physical activity and PTSD. Physical activity as part of an active lifestyle would have the possibility to decrease symptoms of PTSS and PTSD especially in parents of children affected by cancer.

The *integrative model of pediatric medical traumatic stress (PMTS)* can be used as a guide for assessment and intervention for pediatric cancer patients and their families (Kazak et al., 2006). In this context, PMTS and PTSD terms are somewhat interchangeable. The model is divided into three phases, all of which may produce considerable trauma for families. The first phase includes the idea that the child might have a life-threatening condition that is associated with the diagnosis of cancer. The second phase includes demands and challenges from the medical condition itself and the treatments. The last phase addresses persistent traumatic reactions as long-term consequences of the traumatic journey through cancer like and/or the fear of recurrence. The model allows for guidance from professional staff in recognizing trauma in a medical setting and determining management where potentially physical activity could be beneficial.

Pediatric Oncology Patients

Despite studies revealing that parents have higher rates of PTSD following the diagnosis of a severe chronic illness, children may also present with symptoms of post-traumatic stress disorder from their experience with cancer (Landolt et al., 2003). PTSD symptoms are present among 2–20% of children cancer survivors (Taieb, Moro, Baubet, Revah-Levy, & Flament, 2003). Childhood cancer accounts for less than 1% of all new cancer diagnoses in Canada (Canadian Cancer Society's Advisory Committee on Cancer Statistics, 2017). According to the Canadian Cancer Society website (December 12, 2016), between 2009 and 2013, there were 4715 new cases of cancer in children 0–14 years of age in Canada, an average of 943 cases per year, and between 2008 and 2012, there were 595 cancer deaths in the same age group, an average of 119 deaths per year. Death by cancer is the second leading cause of death in Canadian children after accident-related deaths (Canadian Cancer Society, 2016). Kids Cancer Care reports that one in five Canadian children with cancer do not survive (Kid Cancer Care, 2017). They also mention that 75% of children who survived cancer will live with permanent side effects like deafness, blindness, growth issues, motor and cognitive impairments, organ damage (heart, kidney), infertility, psychological issues, and neurological and/or endocrine disorders (Kid Cancer Care, 2017). Although cancer incidence in children might seem low (estimated to be 0.7% in 2017 in 0–19 years age group), it will have an impact not only on the children but also on their families (Canadian Cancer Society's Advisory Committee on Cancer Statistics, 2017).

Childhood cancer may be considered a traumatic event although it is not clear what the traumatic stressors are of this illness (Kazak et al., 1998). The DSM-V specifically mentions that a life-threatening illness is not automatically considered a traumatic event compared to what was written in the earlier version of the DSM and that all other criteria also need to be met (American.Psychiatric.Association, 2013). The cancer journey includes many events that may be considered traumatic for the children and their parents. The diagnosis can be traumatic in itself as well as when parents realize that their child is affected by an illness that poses a threat to his/her life even with treatment (Kazak et al., 1998). Treatment procedures are very repetitive and often painful as well as invasive and/or associated with considerable complications (Kazak et al., 1998; Rabineau et al., 2008). Fear and helplessness are usually present in parents of sick children (Kazak et al., 1998; Rabineau et al., 2008). For many parents, the fear of their child relapsing and dying still remains even after treatment (Kazak et al., 1998). All of these reasons may contribute to post-traumatic stress symptoms among parents.

A systematic review conducted in 2006 mentioned demographic factors that might contribute to the development of PTSD\PTSS in children such as female gender, younger age, separation from parents before the age of 10, family history of psychological problems, poor parental coping, parental exposure to trauma, maternal preoccupation with trauma, maternal PTSD, and recurrence of trauma (Bruce, 2006). These findings suggest that helping parents cope with PTSD/PTSS might lessen some of the symptoms of PTSD in their children and other complications. Young children who lack life experience rely on adults and their environment to construct their reactions and response to situations creating a stronger and more probable association between parental PTSD and child PTSD (Landolt et al., 2003). Stress in parents can negatively impact the support they can provide to their child and the child's social, emotional, and behavioral adjustment to the diagnosis and treatment of cancer (Rabineau et al., 2008).

Parents of Pediatric Oncology Patients

Parents of pediatric cancer patients suffer many challenges and can demonstrate symptoms of post-traumatic stress disorder. A prevalence of 10–44% of severe PTSS and 27–54% prevalence of lifetime PTSD was found in parents of child with cancer (Bruce, 2006). The review by Bruce (2006) reported higher rates of post-traumatic stress in parents than in their child. It is thought that parents experience more symptoms of PTSD than their children because they are traumatized by their own experiences, such as the feeling of guilt and their child experiences related to cancer (Landolt et al., 2003). Other than the trauma that can be caused by the diagnosis in itself, parents have to watch their child experience multiple and difficult treatments, provide informed consent, worry about the side effects, and experience economic and time constraint burdens as a consequence of the illness (Barr & Sala, 2003; Landolt et al., 2003; Nakayama et al., 2016). At the end of the treatment, parents may experience long-term stressors associated with cancer. They often live in fear of late-appearing side-effects of cancer and the fear of disease recurrence (Nakayama et al., 2016). Gender differences were detected in 39.7% of mothers and 33.3% of fathers of childhood cancer survivors (Stuber, Christakis, Houskamp, & Kazak, 1996). Another similar study found that 68% of mothers and 57% of fathers suffered from moderate to severe PTSS according to the PTSD reaction index (PTSD-RI) (Kazak et al., 2005). It seems that over the years, the percentage of parents showing PTSS symptoms have been increasing.

Nakayama et al. (2016) came to the conclusion that parents of children with cancer who have higher trait anxiety may experience chronic anxiety, which may inhibit the cognitive and emotional processes leading to post-traumatic growth (PTG). PTG was defined as "positive psychological change experienced as a result of the struggle with highly challenging life circumstances" (Nakayama et al., 2016). In the same study, it was suggested that the anxiety problem should be dealt with before addressing PTG. A strong association was found between trait anxiety and PTSS suggesting that trait anxiety is a good predictor of adjustment regarding traumatic events (Kazak et al., 1998). Other factors have been found to increase the risk of developing PTSD and/or showing PTSS among parents including variables such as lower level of intelligence, younger age, female gender, social economic status, social support, personality and cognitive features (neuroticism), catastrophic appraisal of trauma, external locus of control, and avoidant coping (Bruce, 2006).

Parents that are separated, divorced, or widowed are also more at risk of developing PTSD (Van Ameringen et al., 2008). Social support plays an important role in the prevention of PTSD (Kazak et al., 1998).

Physical Activity as an Important Intervention

Physical activity may act as primary and secondary prevention of severe chronic diseases and premature death (Warburton, Nicol, & Bredin, 2006). Chronic diseases include mainly cancer, diabetes, obesity, hypertension, osteoarthritis, and depression. Among all the modifiable risk factors for chronic diseases, physical inactivity is the highest modifiable risk factor in 51% of the Canadian population (Warburton et al., 2006).

Physical Fitness in Canada

Examining the physical fitness of the population of adults in Canada between 2012 and 2013, only one in five Canadian adults met the recommended Canadian Physical Activity Guidelines for adults of 150 minutes of moderate physical activity per week according to a publication by Statistics Canada (Ellison, Lawrence, & Janz, 2015). The same publication also reported that between the ages of 18 and 39, 32% met the recommendations, and only 18% did between the ages of 40 and 59 (Ellison et al., 2015). Examples of daily life physical activities can be categorized into occupational, sports, conditioning, household, or leisure activities which include walking, running, biking, swimming, and so forth (Caspersen et al., 1985). The prevalence of suboptimal fitness levels has increased significantly between 1981 and 2009 (Shields et al., 2010). This suggests that the adult Canadians are not doing enough physical activity, and if the trend continues, time allowed to do physical activity will continue to decrease.

Parents of children with cancer can see their own health declining. Common symptoms they experience are fatigue, weight change, and increased blood pressure as well as psychosocial functioning impairment, suicidal ideation, and substance abusive behavior tendencies (Rabineau et al., 2008; Rosenbaum, Vancampfort, et al., 2015). There is evidence that individuals with PTSD have a 2–3 times greater risk of premature death compared to the general population, due to cardiovascular disease (CVD) and metabolic disease which are commonly associated with PTSD (Vancampfort et al., 2016). Physical activity is known to reduce risk of morbidity and mortality in the presence of cardiovascular and metabolic diseases in helping to control blood pressure, lipid levels, and diabetes (Hall et al., 2015). A person who follows an exercise regimen will have improved sleep, and it may engender mastery meaning that it will reinforce adaptive beliefs that parents are in control of their environment to achieve desirable outcomes (Asmundson et al., 2013).

Physical Activity and PTSD

Physical activity and its beneficial impact on mental health such as anxiety and depression disorders have been studied (Asmundson et al., 2013; Cooney et al., 2013; Jayakody, Gunadasa, & Hosker, 2014), but little research has evaluated the impact of physical activity on PTSD until recently. It is hypothesized that physical activity would have a beneficial impact on PTSD (Hall et al., 2015). Two randomized controlled trials were published in 2015 stating the benefits of physical activity on PTSD (Fetzner & Asmundson, 2015; Rosenbaum, Sherrington, & Tiedemann, 2015). Aerobic exercise was found to have therapeutic benefits in individual with PTSD, anxiety, and depression (Fetzner & Asmundson, 2015). One month after the start of the trial, during the study of Fetzner and Asmundson (2015), 86.7% of the participants presented with a reduction in their PCL-C score. PCL-C is a 17-item PTSD civilian checklist that assesses post-traumatic stress symptoms according to the diagnostic criteria of PTSD established by the American Psychiatric Association (Weathers et al., 2013). Another RTC used the same method to analyze the impact of a combined resistant-training and walking program on PTSD symptoms in addition to usual pharmaceutical care (Rosenbaum et al., 2015). Results showed a reduction in PTSS beyond usual care alone and a reduction in depression symptoms and metabolic risk as well (Rosenbaum et al., 2015). These studies provide evidence that physical activity should be included in PTSD care as adjunctive treatment. Any physical activity is more effective at decreasing PTSD than any sedentary conditions (Rosenbaum, Vancampfort, et al., 2015). Physical activity on its own seems to be efficacious at reducing PTSS compared to usual care, but the evidence is limited (Rosenbaum, Vancampfort, et al., 2015). It was also found that physical activity helps improve the mental health of individual with PTSD by providing physiological resilience to stressful mood (Asmundson et al., 2013). Finally, physical activity allows for social interaction and breaks the isolation pattern often present in parents of children with cancer. With all this evidence, physical activity has proven to be an efficacious treatment for patient with anxiety disorder and PTSD (Asmundson et al., 2013), and parents of pediatrics patients would most likely benefit from adding an exercise or sport routine in their everyday life as treatment and/or prevention of PTSS.

Discussion

The main goal of this literature review was to explore the possibility and relevance of including physical activity as an important intervention in the management of PTSD in parents of pediatric oncology patients. In assessing the relationship between physical activity and PTSD, the literature suggests that there are multiple events in the cancer journey that can be traumatic (i.e., diagnosis, treatment, relapse, etc.). Evidence shows that fathers and, often more times, mothers were at risk of developing PTSD. Family-based interventions are needed since they can have a beneficial impact across the course of the illness. Currently, the guidelines in the treatment of PTSD include cognitive–behavioral therapy (CBT) and pharmacological therapy (e.g., selective serotonin reuptake inhibitors (SSRIs)). Problem solving skill training was also found efficient in reducing affect in mothers of children newly diagnosed with cancer (Kearney, Salley, & Muriel, 2015). Physical activity has proven to have beneficial effect in improving symptoms of post-traumatic stress as well as decreasing co-morbidities associated with PTSD. These findings suggest that physical activity decreases distress and anxiety, therefore can lead indirectly to promote *post-traumatic growth* in parents of children affected by cancer (Nakayama et al., 2016).

This literature from this review suggests that physical activities are an important intervention for PTSD in parents of pediatric cancer patients; however, certain questions remain. Most of the literature reviewed used the DSM-IV as a reference in recognizing and the diagnosis of PTSD. Changes made to the DSM from version IV to V could affect the validity and the accuracy of the definition and recognized symptoms of PTSD. DSM criteria are hard to apply to cancer. Only one theory, the PMTS, has tried to understand how cancer can be a source of post-traumatic stress. There is still considerable uncertainty around what exactly, as part of the cancer experience, causes post-traumatic stress. Bruce (2006) also questions the causes of PTSD and indicates that the conceptualization of PTSD and PTSS has been poorly articulated due to the associated predictors which vary widely in this population.

Implications for Clinical Practice

Few studies have been found to evaluate the actual cause and effect of exercise on PTSD (Fetzner & Asmundson, 2015), and only one RCT was found to assess the difference between exercise and the usual treatment plan (Rosenbaum et al., 2015). However, the material that was presented in this chapter can inform oncology professionals and health-care providers to better prepare themselves by recognizing and utilizing more effective interventions that address the specific needs of both the parent and their children with PTSD. Public health services should educate the population and health-care providers by promoting awareness of factors that predispose the development of PTSD (Van Ameringen et al., 2008) such as the type and duration of cancer, the type of treatment, and sociodemographic variables. In-service training for hospital oncologists and nurses focusing on the benefits of physical fitness programs should be promoted for those working directly with pediatric cancer patients and their parents. Referrals should be made post-hospitalization to various community cancer centers in which physical activity is included as a necessary and beneficial treatment intervention. In many cases referrals are made by the attending physician, and a treatment plan is devised in coordination with the physical therapist at the center, which will address the abilities of the patient or their family. However, some cancer centers do not service parents of childhood survivors;

however, physical activity is easily accessible in the community and is associated with minimal cost and may prevent waiting for other treatment options (Fetzner & Asmundson, 2015).

Clinicians should encourage and arrange respite services and family support groups for parents who are experiencing considerable stress and isolation while providing daily care and supervision at home for their child's treatment. In addition, creation of support groups for nurses who are also dealing with families affected by cancer might improve care as well. Attempts to identify and address predisposing factors to PTSD could reduce the prevalence of co-morbid conditions and decrease the societal burden that comes with this disorder.

This literature review provided further evidence and support to the relevance and benefits of physical activity in the management of PTSD in parents of pediatric cancer patients. Evidence shows that physical activity has an important role in the multidisciplinary team management of people with PTSD (Rosenbaum, Vancampfort, et al., 2015) by developing guidelines for programs when implementing physical activity in the treatment plan for PTSD. Specific mechanisms which precipitate and maintain PTSD and PTSS in this clinical population should be explored (Bruce, 2006). Many studies covered in this review have included self-reported questionnaires. It would be interesting to see the results of a study using a community sample with face-to-face interviews as a method of assessment. Results are likely to provide further accuracy and precision. PTSD can lead to a severe mental disorder that should be recognized, diagnosed, and treated by health-care professionals in parents with child affected by cancer. Physical activity has the potential to make a positive difference in the management and quality of life in this specific population.

References

American.Psychiatric.Association. (2013). *Diagnostic and statistical manual of mental disorders: DSM-5* (5th ed.). Washington, DC: American Psychiatric Association.

Asmundson, G. J., Fetzner, M. G., Deboer, L. B., Powers, M. B., Otto, M. W., & Smits, J. A. (2013). Let's get physical: A contemporary review of the anxiolytic effects of exercise for anxiety and its disorders. *Depression and Anxiety, 30*(4), 362–373. https://doi.org/10.1002/da.22043

Barr, R. D., & Sala, A. (2003). Hidden financial costs in the treatment for childhood cancer. *Journal of Pediatric Hematology/Oncology, 25*(11), 842–844.

Bruce, M. (2006). A systematic and conceptual review of posttraumatic stress in childhood cancer survivors and their parents. *Clinical Psychology Review, 26*(3), 233–256. https://doi.org/10.1016/j.cpr.2005.10.002

Canadian Cancer Society's Advisory Committee on Cancer Statistics (2017). Canadian Cancer Statistics 2017. Toronto, ON: Canadian Cancer Society. Available at: https://cancer.ca/Canadian-Cancer-Statistics-2017-EN.pdf

Canadian Cancer Society (2016). Childhood Cancer Statistics. Retrieved December 12th, 2016 from http://www.cancer.ca/en/cancer-information/cancer-101/childhood-cancer-statistics/?region=on

Caspersen, C. J., Powell, K. E., & Christenson, G. M. (1985). Physical activity, exercise, and physical fitness: Definitions and distinctions for health-related research. *Public Health Reports, 100*(2), 126–131.

Cooney, G. M., Dwan, K., Greig, C. A., Lawlor, D. A., Rimer, J., Waugh, F. R., ... Mead, G. E. (2013). Exercise for depression. *Cochrane Database of Systematic Reviews, 9*, Cd004366. https://doi.org/10.1002/14651858.CD004366.pub6

Ellison, L., & Janz, T. (2015). Childhood cancer incidence and mortality in Canada. *Health at a Glance*. Ottawa, ON: Statistic Canada.

Fetzner, M. G., & Asmundson, G. J. (2015). Aerobic exercise reduces symptoms of posttraumatic stress disorder: A randomized controlled trial. *Cognitive Behaviour Therapy, 44*(4), 301–313. https://doi.org/10.1080/16506073.2014.916745

Hall, K. S., Hoerster, K. D., & Yancy, W. S., Jr. (2015). Post-traumatic stress disorder, physical activity, and eating behaviors. *Epidemiologic Reviews, 37*, 103–115. https://doi.org/10.1093/epirev/mxu011

Hoven, E., Gronqvist, H., Poder, U., von Essen, L., & Lindahl Norberg, A. (2017). Impact of a child's cancer disease on parents' everyday life: A longitudinal study from Sweden. *Acta Oncologica, 56*(1), 93–100. https://doi.org/10.1080/0284186x.2016.1250945

Jayakody, K., Gunadasa, S., & Hosker, C. (2014). Exercise for anxiety disorders: Systematic review. *British Journal of Sports Medicine, 48*(3), 187–196. https://doi.org/10.1136/bjsports-2012-091287

Kazak, A. E., Boeving, C. A., Alderfer, M. A., Hwang, W. T., & Reilly, A. (2005). Posttraumatic stress symptoms during treatment in parents of children with cancer. *Journal of Clinical Oncology, 23*(30), 7405–7410. https://doi.org/10.1200/jco.2005.09.110

Kazak, A. E., Kassam-Adams, N., Schneider, S., Zelikovsky, N., Alderfer, M. A., & Rourke, M. (2006). An integrative model of pediatric medical traumatic stress. *Journal of Pediatric Psychology, 31*(4), 343–355. https://doi.org/10.1093/jpepsy/jsj054

Kazak, A. E., Stuber, M. L., Barakat, L. P., Meeske, K., Guthrie, D., & Meadows, A. T. (1998). Predicting posttraumatic stress symptoms in mothers and fathers of survivors of childhood cancers. *Journal of the American Academy of Child and Adolescent Psychiatry, 37*(8), 823–831. https://doi.org/10.1097/00004583-199808000-00012

Kearney, J. A., Salley, C. G., & Muriel, A. C. (2015). Standards of psychosocial care for parents of children with cancer. *Pediatric Blood & Cancer, 62*(Suppl 5), S632–S683. https://doi.org/10.1002/pbc.25761

Kid Cancer Care. (2017). Stats- Kids Cancer Care. Retrieved from www.kidscancercare.ab.ca/childhood-cancer/stats

Landolt, M. A., Vollrath, M., Ribi, K., Gnehm, H. E., & Sennhauser, F. H. (2003). Incidence and associations of parental and child posttraumatic stress symptoms in pediatric patients. *Journal of Child Psychology and Psychiatry, 44*(8), 1199–1207.

Leimanis, M. L., & Fitzpatrick, T. R. (2014). Physical activities and distress among participants of a Cancer Wellness Centre: A community-based pilot study. *International Journal of Physical Medicine & Rehabilitation, 2*, 193. https://doi.org/10.4172/2329-9096.1000193

Ljungman, L., Cernvall, M., Gronqvist, H., Ljotsson, B., Ljungman, G., & von Essen, L. (2014). Long-term positive and negative psychological late effects for parents of childhood cancer survivors: A systematic review. *PLoS One, 9*(7), e103340. https://doi.org/10.1371/journal.pone.0103340

Maddox, G. L. (2001). *The Encyclopedia of Aging: A comprehensive resource in gerontology and geriatrics* (3rd ed.). New York, NY: Springer Publishing.

Nakayama, N., Mori, N., Ishimaru, S., Ohyama, W., Yuza, Y., Kaneko, T., ... Matsushima, E. (2016). Factors associated with posttraumatic growth among parents of children with cancer. *Psycho-Oncology*. https://doi.org/10.1002/pon.4307

Powers, M. B., Medina, J. L., Burns, S., Kauffman, B. Y., Monfils, M., Asmundson, G. J., ... Smits, J. A. (2015). Exercise augmentation of exposure therapy for PTSD: Rationale and pilot efficacy data. *Cognitive Behaviour Therapy, 44*(4), 314–327. https://doi.org/10.1080/16506073.2015.1012740

Rabineau, K. M., Mabe, P. A., & Vega, R. A. (2008). Parenting stress in pediatric oncology populations. *Journal of Pediatric Hematology/Oncology, 30*(5), 358–365. https://doi.org/10.1097/MPH.0b013e318168e76b

Rosenbaum, S., Sherrington, C., & Tiedemann, A. (2015). Exercise augmentation compared with usual care for post-traumatic stress disorder: A randomized controlled trial. *Acta Psychiatrica Scandinavica, 131*(5), 350–359. https://doi.org/10.1111/acps.12371

Rosenbaum, S., Vancampfort, D., Steel, Z., Newby, J., Ward, P. B., & Stubbs, B. (2015). Physical activity in the treatment of post-traumatic stress disorder: A systematic review and meta-analysis. *Psychiatry Research, 230*(2), 130–136. https://doi.org/10.1016/j.psychres.2015.10.017

Shields, M., Tremblay, M. S., Laviolette, M., Craig, C. L., Janssen, I., & Connor Gorber, S. (2010). Fitness of Canadian adults: Results from the 2007-2009 Canadian Health Measures Survey. *Health Reports, 21*(1), 21–35.

Stuber, M. L., Christakis, D. A., Houskamp, B., & Kazak, A. E. (1996). Posttrauma symptoms in childhood leukemia survivors and their parents. *Psychosomatics, 37*(3), 254–261. https://doi.org/10.1016/s0033-3182(96)71564-5

Taieb, O., Moro, M. R., Baubet, T., Revah-Levy, A., & Flament, M. F. (2003). Posttraumatic stress symptoms after childhood cancer. *European Child & Adolescent Psychiatry, 12*(6), 255–264. https://doi.org/10.1007/s00787-003-0352-0

Van Ameringen, M., Mancini, C., Patterson, B., & Boyle, M. H. (2008). Post-traumatic stress disorder in Canada. *CNS Neuroscience & Therapeutics, 14*(3), 171–181. https://doi.org/10.1111/j.1755-5949.2008.00049.x

Vancampfort, D., Stubbs, B., Richards, J., Ward, P. B., Firth, J., Schuch, F. B., & Rosenbaum, S. (2016). Physical fitness in people with posttraumatic stress disorder: A systematic review. *Disability and Rehabilitation*, 1–7. https://doi.org/10.1080/09638288.2016.1226412

Warburton, D. E., Nicol, C. W., & Bredin, S. S. (2006). Health benefits of physical activity: The evidence. *CMAJ, 174*(6), 801–809. https://doi.org/10.1503/cmaj.051351

Weathers, F. W., Litz, B. T., Keane, T. M., Palmieri, P. A., Marx, B. P., & Schnurr, P. P. (2013). The PTSD Checklist for DSM-5 (PCL-5). Scale available from the *National Center for PTSD* at www.ptsd.va.gov.

Chapter 10
Theoretical Perspectives of Post-Traumatic Stress Disorder and Quality of Life Among Young Adult Survivors of Childhood Cancer

Fatima Boulmalf and Tanya R. Fitzpatrick

Introduction

Children are particularly vulnerable to the effects of exposure to trauma, whether physical or emotional. In "Children and Trauma: An Update for Mental Health Professionals", a report puclished by the American Psychological Association, a traumatic event is defined as "one that threatens injury, death, or the physical integrity of self or others and also causes horror, terror, or helplessness at the time it occurs (La Greca et al., 2009, p. 2)." Childhood cancer, from diagnosis to treatment and remission, constitutes such an event. The diagnosis itself is a threat to the child's physical integrity and engenders fear and uncertainty. Furthermore, the process of undergoing treatment and testing often interrupts a child's ability to engage in play and disrupts school attendance and other social interactions. Prolonged hospitalizations and the administration of sometimes painful treatments also contribute to a child's suffering. Given the nature of such an experience and the broad spectrum of diagnoses and treatment modalities, an exploration of the presence, or lack thereof, of post-traumatic stress disorder (PTSD) symptoms in survivors of childhood cancer is warranted. Trauma-related symptoms observed in survivors include "avoidant behaviors, intrusive thoughts and heightened arousability" (Bruce, 2006). The purpose of this chapter is to investigate the prevalence of post-traumatic stress disorder symptoms among young adults who were diagnosed with cancer as children. Additional factors include the type of cancer and the treatment modality, as well as the perceived threat, age at diagnosis, gender, and family functioning. With advances in medical technology and therapies,

F. Boulmalf (✉)
McGill University, Montreal, QC, Canada

T. R. Fitzpatrick
Department of Social Work, Arizona State University, Westmount, QC, Canada
e-mail: Tanya.fitzpatrick@asu.edu

T. R. Fitzpatrick (ed.), *Quality of Life Among Cancer Survivors*,
https://doi.org/10.1007/978-3-319-75223-5_10

increasing numbers of children survive cancer (Bruce, 2006; Tremolada, Bonichini, Basso, & Pillon, 2016). However, these children seldom receive sustained psychological care and support in the subsequent years. Psychological sequelae of childhood cancer may take years to manifest, and absence of care may result in poorer outcomes. Gaining a better understanding of the effect of childhood cancer on a child's growth and mental health years down the line may inform decisions regarding the care that must be provided to children who survive cancer as they proceed with their transition into early adulthood.

If the prevalence of PTSD symptoms among young adult survivors of childhood cancer is significantly higher than in the general population, this may signal a need for the allocation of resources for psychological care and support for children undergoing treatment and in the years following (Tremolada et al., 2016). Furthermore, a correlation between a treatment modality and a higher prevalence of PTSD symptoms may influence choice of treatment when there isn't a definite indication for a modality. Recognizing potential risks and resilience factors may help health-care workers monitor and moderate modifiable variables. PTSD symptoms are associated with reduced subjective quality of life, and this negative correlation has been demonstrated in both cross-sectional and longitudinal studies (Giacco, Matanov, & Priebe, 2013). Therefore, the importance of this chapter lies in the fact that working toward mitigating or preventing onset of these PTSD symptoms in survivors of childhood cancer will lead to improvements in subjective quality of life.

Theoretical Perspectives

The relationship between childhood cancer and the development of post-traumatic stress symptoms in young adulthood has been examined within a framework of the *diathesis-stress model.* This model posits that "traumatic events function as stressors that interact with vulnerabilities to influence the development of PTSD" (Elwood, Mott, Williams, Lohr, & Schroeder, 2009, p. 544). Per this model, stressor events are primary activators of PTSD, but pre-trauma individual differences are important contributing factors. It therefore follows that "individuals who possess higher levels of psychological vulnerabilities before the traumatic experience are at a higher risk for the development of PTSD" (Elwood et al., 2009, p. 545). If a causality can be established between preexisting vulnerabilities and the development of post-traumatic stress symptoms, this can have important implications for prevention and treatment of PTSD, as the diathesis-stress model proposes that vulnerability factors also play a role in the maintenance of symptoms (Elwood et al., 2009). The concept of *cognitive vulnerability* emerged from this model, and cognitive theories were developed, notably the *shattered assumptions* theory, which proposes that a traumatic event *shatters* an individual's established worldview and perception of self and that the experience renders it quasi-impossible for the individual to reconcile pre-trauma beliefs with the new reality (Janoff-Bulman, 1992). Perceptions of control and stability are disrupted by traumatic events, and the *psychological buffering* of the pre-trauma worldview, namely, the belief in "a just, benevolent, predictable world in which the individual possesses competence and worth", is undermined (Edmondson et al., 2011, p. 1).

Similarly, the *terror management theory* suggests that individuals' world views are protective and impart a sense of meaning, purpose, and invulnerability (Pyszczynski, Greenberg, & Solomon, 1999). The theory proposes a *psychological conflict* between the desire to live and awareness of one's mortality and posits that "human awareness of the inevitability of death exerts a profound influence on diverse aspects of human thought, emotion, motivation, and behavior" (Pyszczynski, Solomon, & Greenberg, 2015, p. 2). The *anxiety disruption buffer theory* is an extension of the terror management theory, as "one of the most straightforward implications of TMT is that if a psychological structure serves an anxiety-buffering function, then increasing the strength of that entity should reduce anxiety in threatening situations" (Olson & Zanna, 2015, p. 9). Edmondson et al. (2011) tested the degree to which anxiety buffer parameters are disrupted in individuals who report clinically significant trauma symptoms. The results indicated compromised worldview functioning in individuals with significant trauma symptoms and revealed an inverse relationship between the degree of trauma symptoms and worldview functioning indicators such as self-esteem and meaning, implying impaired anxiety buffer functioning in individuals exhibiting trauma symptoms (Edmondson et al., 2011).

The *hopelessness theory* is one of the most prominent cognitive models of depression and has been employed extensively in the study of depression and cognitive vulnerability since its publication in 1989 by Abramson and colleagues (Liu, Kleiman, Nestor, et al., 2015). The hopelessness theory was initially a reformulation of the *learned helplessness hypothesis*, which postulates that "repeated exposure to uncontrollable and aversive environmental stimuli leads gradually to the belief that the aversive situation is inescapable and a sense of helplessness ensues regarding the situation" and that this sense of helplessness results in depression (Liu et al., 2015, p. 2). The learned helplessness theory did not explain, however, why the same stressors result in depression in some individuals and not others. The hopelessness theory was based on the premise of *negative attributional style* being a predictor of the development of psychopathologies like depression and PTSD. Abramson and colleagues hypothesized that "individuals form causal attributions along three different dimensions, from internal to external, stable to unstable, and from global to specific" and individuals who attribute negative events to internal, stable, and global causes are more susceptible to developing depression (Liu et al., 2015, p. 2). The association of negative attributional style with depression, supported by studies demonstrating increased frequency and severity of depressive symptoms, was then extended to include post-traumatic stress symptoms (Elwood et al., 2009, p. 546).

The concept of *anxiety sensitivity*, or *trait anxiety*, is concordant with the *cognitive vulnerability model* and describes a "stable, trait-like characteristic that functions as a vulnerability to the development and maintenance of anxious symptoms," which precipitates and maintains symptoms of PTSD (Elwood et al., 2009, p. 546). Therefore, not only does anxiety sensitivity predispose an individual to PTSD, but the anxiety prompted by the development of symptoms amplifies the feelings of fear and the need to avoid stimuli perceived as threatening, thus effectively exacerbating the panic symptomatology of PTSD (Fedroff, Taylor, Asmundson, et al., 2000). This theory has been supported by consistent findings of a strong association between anxiety sensitivity and PTSD symptoms and higher levels of reported anxiety sensitivity in PTSD groups compared to non-PTSD groups, establishing anxiety sensitivity as a predictor of PTSD (Elwood et al., 2009).

The *social causation* and *social erosion* hypotheses are two models that are alternately used to interpret the relationship between social support and PTSD. Shallcross and colleagues tested these competing models by conducting separate analyses on measures of perceived social support and PTSD components of intrusion, avoidance, hyper-arousal, and dysphoria, as well as overall PTSD symptoms, and obtained results that supported both models, thus suggesting that "PTSD-specific symptom dimensions may both erode and be influenced by social support, whereas general psychological distress erodes social support" (Shallcross, Arbisi, Polusny, Kramer, & Erbes, 2016, p. 167). *Social causation* infers that lack of social support predisposes individuals to PTSD symptomatology. This model is based on "the fundamental assumption that support resources are critical antecedents of well-being, and a lack of social support precedes, and contributes to, increases in psychological distress" (Shallcross et al., 2016, p. 167). *Social erosion*, on the other hand, theorizes that "social support is itself determined by mental health and distress" (p. 167). The *social erosion hypothesis* is also referred to as *social selection*, as the supposition is that individuals are *selected*, or more importantly *not selected*, for inclusion in social groups based on determinants like mental health and overall well-being. Kaniasty and Norris (2008) summarize this concept aptly:

> In the domain of social support, social selection means that healthy individuals are selected (or welcomed) into thriving social relationships. Conversely, persons with psychological distress may experience a decline in their social support resources. (p. 274)

The *drift hypothesis* is analogous to the social erosion/social selection hypothesis in that it emphasizes the effect of mental illness on the individual's social relationships and ultimately the individual's downward shift in socioeconomic strata. Untethered to strong social relationships and forced to endure loss of income due to their illness, individuals experience a marked downward social mobility. In fact, "the inverse relationship between social class and the occurrence of mental disorders is one of the most well established in the field of mental health epidemiology" (Perry, 1996, p. 17). Goldberg and Morrison (1963) conducted a study to examine the effect of schizophrenia on patients' socioeconomic status and documented a "drift toward inactivity" as they observed that "Slowly their occupational status worsen[ed] and the breadth and mixture of jobs shrink[ed] continually" (p. 796). The study also examined the distribution of the fathers of schizophrenic patients by occupation and found a normal distribution; however, the authors note that "the finding that the fathers of schizophrenic patients represent a typical occupational cross section of the community in which they live and that they have, on the whole, steady and solid work careers, does not imply that they are particularly well adjusted in other respects; that family relationships were undisturbed or, in particular, that their relations with their sick sons were positive" (Goldberg & Morrison, 1963, p. 798).

Gender and Trauma

Being female is often positioned as a putative risk factor for PTSS in childhood cancer survivors, and its association with trauma-related symptomatology is meticulously analyzed. This is to be expected given the long history of research regarding gender and trauma. In a quantitative review of 25 years of research on sex differences in trauma and PTSD, a twofold risk of PTSD among female participants compared with male participants was observed (Tolin & Foa, 2006). In this study, a meta-analysis of sex differences in the prevalence of potentially traumatic events (PTE) revealed that male participants were significantly more likely to report a PTE than female participants. It was hypothesized that "compared with male participants, female participants are more likely to experience certain types of PTE that are disproportionately likely to lead to PTSD" (p. 964). Tolin and Foa (2006) concluded their analysis as follows:

> With regard to the question of whether female participants are more likely than male participants to meet diagnostic criteria for PTSD, we found that regardless of the type of study, population, type of assessment, or other methodological variables, women and girls are more likely than men and boys to meet criteria for PTSD. This is consistent with epidemiological research showing a higher prevalence of fear- and anxiety-based disorders in general among female respondents. (p. 977)

In regard to young adult survivors of childhood cancer, numerous studies have confirmed female gender as a strong predictor of PTSS (Hobbie et al., 2000; Kamibeppu et al., 2015; Langeveld et al., 2004; Tremolada et al., 2016). In a study aimed at identifying factors associated with post-traumatic stress symptoms among 185 young adult Japanese childhood cancer survivors, multiple regression analysis revealed an association between being female and an increased risk of PTSS (Kamibeppu et al., 2015). These findings are consistent with the portrait of PTSD in the general population, as "one of the most consistent findings in the epidemiology of post-traumatic stress disorder (PTSD) is the higher risk of this disorder in women" (Olff, Langeland, Draijer, & Gersons, 2007, p. 183). Kamibeppu et al. (2015) found that "although being female, older at the time of diagnosis, and having late effects emerged as risk factors for PTSS, symptoms were maintained at low levels if family functioning was high" (p. 539). This observation suggests that family functioning also plays an important role in predicting post-traumatic stress symptoms, which will be discussed in the next section.

Family Functioning and Perceived Social Support

The inverse association between perceived social support and PTSD has been documented extensively in trauma research (Brewin, Andrews, & Valentine, 2000; Clapp & Beck, 2009; Ozer, Best, Lipsey, & Weiss, 2003). Furthermore, the literature on social support suggests that individuals' perceptions of their social networks and the support offered to them by these networks play a role in whether these individuals seek out and make use of social resources (Tolsdorf, 1976). The results that have solidified the association between PTSD and social support, for example, the meta-analysis conducted by Ozer et al. (2003), have been interpreted within the framework of the *stress-buffering model*, which was elaborated by Cohen and Wills in 1985 (Clapp & Beck, 2009). In their article, Cohen and Wills sought to determine whether the association between social support and overall well-being is attributable to the overall benefit derived from the support (direct model) or the process of the support protecting individuals from the effects of stressful experiences (buffering model) (Cohen & Wills, 1985). The *direct effect model* implies that the positive effect of social support on well-being is derived irrespective of whether the individual is under stress, whereas the buffering model implies a protective effect; the "theoretical and practical implications" of these processes on the design of interventions are what led Cohen and Wills (1985) to analyze the evidence supporting each theory (p. 313). Although the buffering model is not specific to traumatic stress as such, the premise of the stress-buffering model is that support offered by one's social networks helps the individual cope with stressful events and "buffer against the development of stress-related psychopathology" (Clapp & Beck, 2009, p. 2).

In light of the aforementioned, many studies evaluating the predicting factors of post-traumatic symptoms in young adult survivors of childhood cancer include social support and family functioning as potential contributing factors. In the study conducted by Kamibeppu et al. (2015), family functioning was determined to be "the strongest predictor among several factors found to be associated with PTSS" (p. 539). Tremolada et al. (2016) used the Multidimensional Scale of Perceived Social Support (MSPSS) to measure the "instrumental and emotional social support provided by family, friends, and significant others" (p. 5). The results of this study identified global perceived social support reported by the former patients as an important modifiable predictor of PTSS; single relationship status was associated with higher risk of avoidance symptoms, suggesting that "fewer relationships with others impacted negatively on psychological wellbeing" (Tremolada et al., 2016, p. 6).

In a study aimed primarily at investigating family functioning as well as the relationship between family functioning and post-traumatic stress disorder in young adolescent survivors of childhood cancer, Alderfer, Navsaria, and Kazak (2009) administered a structured diagnostic interview to 144 adolescent cancer survivors (1–12 years post-cancer treatment) and instructed all 144 participants and their parents to complete a Family Assessment Device. The results indicated that 47% of the adolescents, 25% of the mothers, and 30% of the fathers reported poor family functioning; family functioning was poorer in families in which the adolescent cancer survivor met PTSD diagnostic criteria (8%) and three-fourths of the adolescents with PTSD belonged to families with low family functioning scores, making adolescents with PTSD five times more likely to be emerge from a poorly functioning family (p. 1). The authors concluded that family functioning plays a role in traumatic stress reactions of adolescent childhood cancer survivors (Alderfer, Navsaria, & Kazak, 2009). Although this study pertained strictly to the potentially traumatic experience of childhood cancer, the trauma literature suggests that family functioning plays a role across a range of traumatic events (Meiser-Stedman, Yule, Dalgleish, et al., 2006).

Treatment Type and Intensity

Several studies examining the relationship between childhood cancer and PTSD in young adults have also investigated the effect of treatment type and intensity on frequency and severity of post-traumatic stress symptoms, yielding inconsistent results (Brown, Madan-Swain, & Lambert, 2003; Kamibeppu et al., 2015; Rourke, Hobbie, Schwartz, et al., 2007). Brown et al. (2003) computed a disease severity index using medical records, and the average of two independent ratings, one provided by each survivor's primary oncologist and the other provided by another oncologist familiar with the diagnosis and treatment, found that "severity of disease (i.e., number of medical late effects) accounted for a marginally significant portion of the variance in PTSD symptoms for survivors (9%)" (Brown et al., 2003, p. 316). Rourke et al. (2007) examined severable variables relating to treatment and disease, notably diagnosis, time of treatment, and intensity of treatment and severity of medical late effects assessed by the provider. To quantify treatment intensity, the Intensity of Treatment Rating Scale was employed, "rat[ing] the intensity of the cancer treatment protocols based on Children's Oncology Group (COG) protocol number, medications, and treatment modalities" (Rourke et al., 2007, p. 178). The assessment of intensity for each patient was conducted blindly and independently by a pediatric oncologist and a pediatric oncology nurse practitioner, and the raters convened and agreed on a rating in cases where their original assessments were incongruous; data on medical late effects were assessed and rated by the same oncologist and nurse practitioner (Rourke et al., 2007). The results of this study revealed no significant difference between the two groups (survivors with and without PTSD) in terms of objective measurements of treatment intensity, leading the authors to note that "although more intensive treatment protocols might result in more "exposure" to traumatic events (e.g., more intensive treatments, more hospitalizations, and emergency clinic visits or admissions), the findings highlight the important of subjective appraisals of life events as more predictive of distress than objective medical criteria" (Rourke et al., 2007, p. 181). A different study conducted by Kamibeppu and colleagues (2015) did not find a significant association between treatment intensity, as evaluated by the second version of the Intensity of

Treatment Rating Scale (ITR-2), and post-traumatic stress symptoms and also suggested that the perceived treatment intensity, "rather than treatment modalities or objective treatment intensity," may be associated with PTSS (Kamibeppu et al., 2015, p. 540).

Post-Traumatic Growth

In recent years, investigations of PTSS among young adult survivors of childhood cancer have begun to consider the concept of personal growth resulting from trauma and its association with post-traumatic stress symptoms (Klosky et al., 2014). *Post-traumatic growth*, or PTG, "refers to the positive changes resulting from the struggle with a traumatic event, and not to the changes caused by the event itself," and has been used interchangeable with the concept of *benefit finding* (Klosky et al., 2014, p. 879). Benefit finding is defined as "the process of deriving positive growth from adversity" and has been a key concept in the development of the positive psychology approach (Cassidy, McLaughlin, & Giles, 2014, p. 268). For there to be post-traumatic growth, the traumatic event must have been sufficiently stressful to "challenge the individual's worldview and precipitate a rethinking or reordering of priorities" (Klosky et al., 2014, p. 879). This is comparable to the *shattered assumptions theory* in that the traumatic event is considered to constitute a disruption to the individual's pre-trauma perspective. The Post-traumatic Growth Inventory is used to assess post-traumatic growth through five different components (relating to others, new possibilities, personal strength, spiritual change, and appreciation of life) and generates a total score, in which a higher score delineates greater post-traumatic growth (Klosky et al., 2014). This score was used by Klosky et al. (2014) to evaluate the association between post-traumatic growth and post-traumatic stress symptoms, with results "suggesting a weak, but positive, relationship between these two constructs" (p. 880). A different study evaluating post-traumatic growth and post-traumatic stress symptoms in 223 childhood cancer survivors identified "significant associations between PTG and PTSS" (Tremolada et al., 2016, p. 5).

Yi and Kim (2014) used the Post-traumatic Growth Inventory (PTGO) and the Post-traumatic Stress Diagnostic Scale (PDS) to analyze the relationship between post-traumatic stress and post-traumatic growth and found that "PDS was negatively associated with the total PTGI" with greater levels of PDS related to lower levels of PTGI (p. 464). Yi and Kim (2014) evoked the *stress theory* (recall the diathesis-stress theory) as a potential explanation for these findings, given that the stress theory proposes that post-traumatic stress is detrimental to human functioning and quality of life and thus "cannot be linked to growth experiences" (p. 464). In an exploration of post-traumatic growth in cancer specifically, Sumalla, Ochoa, and Blanco (2009) surmised that "the characteristics of cancer, such as the difficulty in identifying a sole stressor, the internal nature of the illness, the temporal orientation with the subject's fears focused on the future as well as obvious traumatic memories, the practical impossibility of establishing the onset and termination of the traumatic event, together with differences in perceived control, all justify the differential clinical setting of cancer as a chronic extreme stressor" (p. 32). Therefore, the fundamental differences between cancer and other kinds of trauma may explain the negative, linear PTSD/PTG relationship observed in this study (Yi & Kim, 2014).

Age at Diagnosis

It is often hypothesized that a younger age at diagnosis of cancer is a risk factor for the development of PTSD, and many studies investigating the prevalence of post-traumatic stress symptoms in young adult survivors of childhood cancer have put this assumption to the test (Tremolada et al., 2016; Rourke et al., 2007; Kunin-Batson et al., 2011; Klosky et al., 2014; etc.). In their study, Kamibeppu and colleagues (2015) obtained a significant association between the interaction of age at diagnosis with family function and PTSS. Rourke et al. (2007) established age at diagnosis as a significant predictor of PTSD in a model combining trait anxiety, female gender, and other variables related to the individual's subjective perceptions of the impact of cancer (intensity, life threat, etc.), with this model yielding an overall success rate of 89.4% (p. 180). Rourke et al. (2007) stipulate, however, that "odds ratios for the significant predictors are small[,] indicating small changes in the likelihood of a PTSD diagnosis with a one-unit change in each variable" (p. 180). Yi and Kim (2014), while investigating the relationship between post-traumatic stress and post-traumatic growth in childhood cancer survivors, found that "older age and shorter time since diagnosis were associated with the higher levels of the total PTGI" (P. 464). This follows their finding of a negative association between PTGI and PTSD, which may suggest that younger age at diagnosis is associated with a higher severity of post-traumatic stress symptoms. Similarly, Klosky and colleagues found that survivors diagnosed at 5 years old and above "were between 1.4 [to] 2.1 times more likely to report increases in PTG" (Klosky et al., 2014, p. 880). In a study evaluating the independent living status of adult survivors of childhood cancer, it was revealed that "survivors who were at least 12 years of age at diagnosis were more than twice as likely to live independently than those diagnosed and treated prior to 6 years of age" (Kunin-Batson et al., 2011, p. 1200).

Prevalence of Post-Traumatic Stress Symptoms

A multitude of studies have demonstrated the prevalence of post-traumatic stress symptomatology in young adult survivors of childhood cancer (Hobbie et al., 2000; Brown et al., 2003; Rourke et al., 2007; Yi & Kim, 2014; Klosky et al., 2014; Kamibeppu et al., 2015; Tremolada et al., 2016). Hobbie and colleagues (2000) assessed 78 young adults aged 18 to 40 years and concluded that one-fifth of the sample of survivors met criteria for PTSD diagnosis. Brown et al. (2003)

found that although none of the participants met DSM-III-R criteria for PTSD diagnosis, "survivors endorsed a greater frequency of stressful life events and PTSD symptoms than their healthy counterparts" (Brown et al., 2003, p. 315). Another study, conducted by Rourke et al. (2007), revealed that 16% of the sample of young adult survivors of childhood cancer met the diagnostic criteria of PTSD (Rourke et al., 2007). Yi and Kim (2014) used a sample of relatively long-term survivors to evaluate the relationship between post-traumatic stress and post-traumatic growth in survivors of childhood cancer. Although none of the survivors met clinically significant levels of post-traumatic stress, 64.3% of the sample reported mild symptoms, and 26.3% reported moderate symptoms. Long-term survivors were recruited in order to allow the evaluation of post-traumatic growth, which may explain these findings given that "the prevalence of PTSD symptoms seems to decline considerably for the majority of survivors 3 months post-diagnosis or following treatment completion" (Yi & Kim, 2014, p. 465). A comparable study performed by Klosky et al. (2014) used a sample of long-term survivors of child cancer to determine the association between post-traumatic stress and post-traumatic growth and reported that over 71% of the participants experience some post-traumatic stress symptoms (Klosky et al., 2014). Kamibeppu and colleagues sought to identify predictors of PTSS among adolescent survivors of childhood cancer and found that 20.7% of the sample had IES-R-J (Impact of Event Scale-Revised; a tool used for evaluation of PTSD criteria) total scores that exceeded the cutoff point for diagnosis of PTSD (Kamibeppu, 2015). Tremolada and colleagues recruited 223 young adult survivors of childhood cancer, 9.4% of whom exhibited clinical PTSD symptomatology and 11.2% subclinical symptomatology (Tremolada et al., 2016, p. 5).

Implications for Subjective Quality of Life (SQOL) and Independence

The association between post-traumatic stress disorder and subjective quality of life has been established empirically, with patients with PTSD consistently reporting a poorer subjective quality of life than those with other anxiety disorders (Giacco et al., 2013). Subjective quality of life is defined as "the patient's satisfaction with life in general and with a number of major life domains" (p. 1). Giacco et al. (2013) documented a progressive and significant improvement of subjective quality of life associated with reduction of PTSD symptoms and discovered a bidirectional association between SQOL and hyperarousal symptoms of PTSD (Giacco et al., 2013). Kunin-Batson and colleagues assessed the independent living status of survivors of childhood cancer and found that "adult survivors of childhood cancer who experience neurocognitive, psychological, or physical late effects are less likely to live independently as adults" (Kunin-Batson et al., 2011, p. 1197). Considering that "a significant subset of young adult survivors of childhood cancer experience symptoms of post-traumatic stress and other psychological difficulties" and that these symptoms have been shown to affect individuals' quality of life and their ability to live independently years down the line, "health care providers can alleviate ongoing cancer-related distress and promote competence" by addressing these issues and anticipating the potential psychological sequelae of childhood cancer survival (Hobbie et al., 2000, p. 4065).

Conclusions

The *diathesis-stress model*, along with the ensuing theories based on *cognitive vulnerability*, succeeds in accounting for both the stressor event and an individual's vulnerability to stress, as determining factors in the development of post-traumatic stress symptoms. It provides a framework for understanding the development of post-traumatic stress symptoms following a traumatic event while allowing for individual variability in regard to vulnerability and predisposition to anxiety and post-traumatic stress. This model allows us to examine the different factors that precipitate the development of symptoms following the experience of childhood cancer. Although to varying degrees, the studies examined for the purpose of this chapter have all confirmed the prevalence of post-traumatic stress symptoms in young adult survivors of childhood cancer. The results suggest that a younger age at diagnosis may be a predictor of greater severity of symptoms, and one study evaluating the independent living status of adult survivors of childhood cancer found a correlation between age at diagnosis and independent living (Kunin-Batson et al., 2011). Furthermore, the different studies examining the relationship between treatment intensity and post-traumatic stress symptoms concluded that perceived, or subjective, treatment intensity plays a more important role in influencing severity of symptoms than the treatment intensity measured with the use of objective medical criteria (Kamibeppu et al., 2015; Rourke et al., 2007).

The *social causation* and *social erosion* models seem to accurately interpret the complex dynamic of social support and psychological stress, as there is evidence to support both models. The inverse association between post-traumatic stress symptoms and social support has been reported on extensively. It stands to reason that individuals with less support following a traumatic experience would fare worse than their counterparts with adequate support and resources available to them. This has been confirmed by Ozer and colleagues (2003) in a meta-analytic study. In their study evaluating the prevalence of post-traumatic symptoms in young adult survivors of childhood cancer, Kamibeppu et al. (2015) propose social support and family functioning as potential contributing factors and find family functioning to be "the strongest predictor" of symptoms. Other studies examining this factor reached similar conclusions (Alderfer, Navsaria, & Kazak, 2009; Tremolada et al., 2016).

The studies reviewed overwhelmingly demonstrate a higher prevalence of post-traumatic stress symptoms among young adult survivors of childhood cancer (Hobbie et al., 2000; Brown et al., 2003; Rourke et al., 2007; Yi & Kim, 2014;

Klosky et al., 2014; Kamibeppu et al., 2015; Tremolada et al., 2016). This has serious implications for the quality of life of survivors, given the demonstrated association between post-traumatic stress and poorer subjective quality of life (Giacco et al., 2013). The aforementioned results and their implications on subjective quality of life can inform health policy makers and health-care professionals in regard to the prevention and treatment of post-traumatic stress symptoms with the ultimate goal of improving survivors' subjective quality of life.

References

Alderfer, M. A., Navsaria, N., & Kazak, A. E. (2009). Family functioning and post-traumatic stress disorder in adolescent survivors of childhood cancer. *Journal of Family Psychology: JFP: Journal of the Division of Family Psychology of the American Psychological Association (Division 43)*, *23*(5), 717–725. https://doi.org/10.1037/a0015996

Brewin, C. R., Andrews, B., & Valentine, J. D. (2000, January 01). Meta-analysis of risk factors for posttraumatic stress disorder in trauma-exposed adults. *Journal of Consulting and Clinical Psychology, 68*, 5, 748–66.

Brown, R. T., Madan-Swain, A., & Lambert, R. (2003, August 01). Post-traumatic stress symptoms in adolescent survivors of childhood cancer and their mothers. *Journal of Traumatic Stress*, *16*(4), 309–318.

Bruce, M. (2006, January 01). A systematic and conceptual review of post-traumatic stress in childhood cancer survivors and their parents. *Clinical Psychology Review*, *26*(3), 233–256.

Cassidy, T., McLaughlin, M., & Giles, M. (2014). Benefit finding in response to general life stress: Measurement and correlates. *Health Psychology and Behavioral Medicine*, *2*(1), 268–282. https://doi.org/10.1080/21642850.2014.889570

Clapp, J. D., & Beck, J. G. (2009). Understanding the relationship between PTSD and social support: The role of negative network orientation. *Behaviour Research and Therapy*, *47*(3), 237–244. https://doi.org/10.1016/j.brat.2008.12.006

Cohen, S., & Wills, T. A. (1985, January 01). Stress, social support, and the buffering hypothesis. *Psychological Bulletin, 98*, 2, 310–57.

Edmondson, D., Chaudoir, S. R., Mills, M. A., Park, C. L., Holub, J., & Bartkowiak, J. M. (2011). From shattered assumptions to weakened world views: Trauma symptoms signal anxiety buffer disruption. *Journal of Loss & Trauma*, *16*(4), 358–385. https://doi.org/10.1080/15325024.2011.572030

Elwood, L. S., Mott, J., Williams, N. L., Lohr, J. M., & Schroeder, D. A. (2009, December 01). Attributional style and anxiety sensitivity as maintenance factors of post-traumatic stress symptoms: A prospective examination of a diathesis-stress model. *Journal of Behavior Therapy and Experimental Psychiatry*, *40*(4), 544–557.

Fedroff, I. C., Taylor, S., Asmundson, G. J. G., & Koch, W. J. (2000, January 01). Cognitive factors in traumatic stress reactions: Predicting PTSD symptoms from anxiety sensitivity and beliefs about harmful events. *Behavioral and Cognitive Psychotherapy*, *28*(1), 5–15.

Giacco, D., Matanov, A., & Priebe, S. (2013). Symptoms and subjective quality of life in post-traumatic stress disorder: A longitudinal study. *PLoS One*, *8*(4), e60991. https://doi.org/10.1371/journal.pone.0060991

Goldberg, E. M., & Morrison, S. L. (1963, January 01). Schizophrenia and social class. *The British Journal of Psychiatry: The Journal of Mental Science*, *109*, 785–802.

Hobbie, W. L., Stuber, M., Meeske, K., Wissler, K., Rourke, M. T., Ruccione, K., Hinkle, A., Kazak, A. E. (2000). Symptoms of posttraumatic stress in young adult survivors of childhood cancer. *Journal of Clinical Oncology, 18*(24), 4060–4066

Janoff-Bulman, R. (1992). *Shattered assumptions: Towards a new psychology of trauma*. New York, NY: Free Press.

Kamibeppu, K., Murayama, S., Ozono, S., Sakamoto, N., Iwai, T., Asami, K., Maeda, N., Inada, H., Kakee, N., Okamura, J., Horibe, K., Ishida, Y. (2015). Predictors of posttraumatic stress symptoms among adolescent and young adult survivors of childhood cancer. *Journal of Family Nursing, 21*(4), 529–550

Kamibeppu, S. (2015). Communication terminal and cancer server and communication system. In US Patent 9185349B2, 185, 349. Google Patent.

Kaniasty, K., & Norris, F. H. (2008, January 01). Longitudinal linkages between perceived social support and post-traumatic stress symptoms: Sequential roles of social causation and social selection. *Journal of Traumatic Stress, 21*(3), 274–281.

Klosky, J. L., Krull, K. R., Kawashima, T., Leisenring, W., Randolph, M. E., Zebrack, B., ... Phipps, S. (2014, January 01). Relations between post-traumatic stress and post-traumatic growth in long-term survivors of childhood cancer: A report from the childhood cancer survivor study. *Health Psychology: Official Journal of the Division of Health Psychology, American Psychological Association, 33*(8), 878–882.

Kunin-Batson, A., Kadan-Lottick, N., Zhu, L., Cox, C., Bordes-Edgar, V., Srivastava, D. K., ... Krull, K. R. (2011). Predictors of independent living status in adult survivors of childhood cancer: A report from the Childhood Cancer Survivor Study. *Pediatric Blood & Cancer, 57*, 1197–1203. https://doi.org/10.1002/pbc.22982

La Greca, A. M., Boyd, B. A., Jaycox, L. H., Kassam-Adams, N., Mannarino, A. P., Silverman, W. K., ... Wong, M., (2009). Children and Trauma. Retrieved Feb 27, 2017, from http://www.apa.org/pi/families/resources/children-trauma-update.aspx

Langeveld, N. E., Grootenhuis, M. A., Voûte, P. A., & de, H. R. J. (2004, June 01). Posttraumatic stress symptoms in adult survivors of childhood cancer. *Pediatric Blood & Cancer, 42*, 7, 604–610.

Liu, R. T., Kleiman, E. M., Nestor, B. A., & Cheek, S. M. (2015). The hopelessness theory of depression: A quarter century in review. *Clinical psychology: A publication of the Division of Clinical Psychology of the American Psychological Association, 22*(4), 345–365. https://doi.org/10.1111/cpsp.12125

Meiser-Stedman, R. A., Yule, W., Dalgleish, T., & Glucksman, E. (2006). The role of the family in child and adolescent post-traumatic stress following attendance at an emergency department. *Journal of Pediatric Psychology, 31*, 397–402. [PubMed: 16606628].

Olff, M., Langeland, W., Draijer, N., & Gersons, B. P. (2007, January 01). Gender differences in posttraumatic stress disorder. *Psychological Bulletin, 133*, 2, 183–204.

Olson, J. M., & Zanna, M. P. (2015). *Advances in experimental social psychology*. Volume 52. Waltham, Massachusetts: Academic Press, an imprint of Elsevier.

Ozer, E. J., Best, S. R., Lipsey, T. L., & Weiss, D. S. (2003, January 01). Predictors of posttraumatic stress disorder and symptoms in adults: a meta-analysis. *Psychological Bulletin, 129*, 1, 52–73.

Perry, M. J. (1996, September 01). The relationship between social class and mental disorder. *Journal of Primary Prevention, 17*(1), 17–30.

Pyszczynski, T., Solomon, S., & Greenberg, J. (2015, January 01). Thirty years of terror management theory: From genesis to revelation. *Advances in Experimental Social Psychology, 52*, 1–70.

Pyszczynski, T., Greenberg, J., Solomon, S. (1999). A duel-process model of defense against conscious and unconscious death-related thoughts: An extension of terror-management theory. *Psychological Review, 106*(4), 835–845.

Rourke, M. T., Hobbie, W. L., Schwartz, L., et al. (2007, August 01). Post-traumatic stress disorder (PTSD) in young adult survivors of childhood cancer. *Pediatric Blood & Cancer, 49*(2), 177–182.

Shallcross, S. L., Arbisi, P. A., Polusny, M. A., Kramer, M. D., & Erbes, C. R. (2016, January 01). Social causation versus social erosion: Comparisons of causal models for relations between support and PTSD symptoms. *Journal of Traumatic Stress, 29*(2), 167–175.

Sumalla, E. C., Ochoa, C., & Blanco, I. (2009, January 01). Post-traumatic growth in cancer: Reality or illusion?. *Clinical Psychology Review, 29*(1), 24–33. https://doi.org/10.1016/j.cpr.2008.09.006

Tolin, D. F., & Foa, E. B. (2006, November 01). Sex differences in trauma and posttraumatic stress disorder: A quantitative review of 25 years of research. *Psychological Bulletin, 132*, 6, 959–992.

Tolsdorf, C. C. (1976). Social networks, support, and coping: An exploratory study. *Family Process, 15*(4), 407–417.

Tremolada, M., Bonichini, S., Basso, G., & Pillon, M. (2016, February 01). Post-traumatic stress symptoms and post-traumatic growth in 223 childhood cancer survivors: Predictive risk factors. *Frontiers in Psychology, 7*.

Yi, J., & Kim, M. A. (2014). Post-cancer experiences of childhood cancer survivors: How is post-traumatic stress related to post-traumatic growth? *Journal of Traumatic Stress, 27*(4), 461–467. https://doi.org/10.1002/jts.21941

Chapter 11
Family Functioning and Therapeutic Interventions When a Parent Has Cancer

Andréa Maria Laizner

Introduction

Healthcare professionals have found it useful to view families from a systems perspective when considering the impact of a cancer diagnosis and treatment on the ill parent and the rest of the family members.

> When viewed as a system, the family can be defined as a complex structure comprised of an interdependent group of individuals who (1) have a shared sense of history; (2) experience some degree of emotional bonding; and (3) devise strategies for meeting the needs of individual family members and the group as a whole. Implicit in the use of the system metaphor to define the family is the premise that the family is structurally complex, is comprised of multiple subsystems, has common purposes and tasks that must be fulfilled, and devise strategies for the execution of these tasks. (Anderson & Sabatelli, 2011, pp. 6)

An important perspective of the family as a system is that the family is more than the sum of its parts and is based on relationships among its parts to function effectively. Added to this is diversity and complexity, which make each family unique. "Knowing who is in the system is important because the composition of the family places demands upon the system and influences interactional patterns" (Anderson & Sabatelli, p. 8). Family functioning is defined as a family's ability to accomplish family tasks through specific processes to meet the needs of both individual family members and wider society (Friedman, Bowden, & Jones, 2003; Walsh, 2012).

A family systems perspective assumes that events are not experienced in isolation but have an impact on other family members. According to Rolland (2005), "the impact of a diagnosis of cancer reverberates throughout the family system, leaving no one untouched" (p. 2584). Having a parent diagnosed with cancer adds to the complexity of family functioning required to keep the family strong. The family unit

A. M. Laizner (✉)
McGill University Health Centre, Nursing Practice Consultant-Research, Nursing Directorate, Montréal, QC, Canada
e-mail: andrea.laizner@muhc.mcgill.ca; andrea.laizner@mcgill.ca

T. R. Fitzpatrick (ed.), *Quality of Life Among Cancer Survivors*,
https://doi.org/10.1007/978-3-319-75223-5_11

can experience major changes in living patterns and routines, roles, and relationships as a consequence of having a parent diagnosed with cancer (Buchbinder, Longhofer, & McCue, 2009; Grabiak, Bender, & Puskar, 2007; Phillips & Lewis, 2015). Therefore many studies initially explored the relationship between family members' psychological adjustment when a parent had cancer (Compas et al., 1994; Phillips, 2014; Purc-Stephensen & Lyseng, 2016). Subsequently, studies began to focus on parental or family functioning and its relationship to psychological adjustment (Osborn, 2007; Phillips, 2014; Schmitt et al., 2008). The research has remained mostly retrospective and cross-sectional with a few prospective studies (Krauel, Simon, Krause-Hebecker, Czimbalmos, Bottomley, & Flechtner, 2012; Osborn, 2007; Phillips, 2014). Although most of the studies were initially with women diagnosed with breast cancer, they eventually included other cancer diagnoses (Fitch, Gray, & Franssen, 2000; Osborn, 2007; Phillips, 2014) and whether the mother or the father was the parent diagnosed with cancer (Osborn, 2007; Phillips, 2014). Family functioning in families with a parent having a limited life expectancy and dependent children was also examined (Kühne et al., 2013).

This chapter will provide further understanding of family functioning when a parent has cancer and its relationship to child and adolescent emotional responses. Strategies for intervention are suggested to address the information and psychological health needs of parents and their children. Implications for healthcare professionals and future research are discussed.

Beginning with Breast Cancer in a Mother to Understand Family System Response

Early research established that breast cancer in the mother was not just experienced by the mother but also by the other family members and the family as a whole (Friedman, Baer, Nelson, Lane, Smith, & Dworkin, 1988; Hilton, 1993a, b, 1994; Hilton & Elfert, 1996; Hilton & Gustavason, 2002; Issel, Ersek, & Lewis, 1990; Lewis & Hammond, 1992; Lewis, Woods, Hough, & Bensley, 1989; Oktay & Walter, 1991; Pederson & Valanis, 1988). There was particular concern for families when the woman was a mother with school-aged or adolescent children (Issel et al., 1990; Lewis & Hammond, 1992; Lewis, Zahlis, Shands, Sinsheimer, & Hammond, 1996; Wellisch, 1981). This was because the patient as parent was expected to cope with the diagnosis, its treatment, and the prognosis while also managing child-rearing and the ongoing demands of maintaining family life.

Husbands reported being distressed for up to 18 months after the diagnosis of breast cancer in a spouse (Maguire, 1981; Northouse, 1990; Northouse, Cracchiolo-Caraway, & Appel, 1993; Northouse & Swain, 1987). Although the marital relationship was often strained when a woman had breast cancer, few ended in divorce (Northouse et al., 1993). Some children and adolescents were reporting difficulty obtaining support within the family (Issel et al., 1990). Adolescent children were developmentally at a point in their lives when they needed to separate from their family of origin, and parents needed to let go and help their children to achieve autonomy (Friedman et al., 2003; Oktay & Walter, 1991; Preto, 1989; Wellisch, 1981). Consequently, mothers with breast cancer, who were dealing with diagnosis and treatment, likely found it difficult to help their children and adolescents and possibly wanted some support from their adolescent children. There was evidence that making such a transition to independence was particularly difficult for adolescent daughters since they often took on more responsibilities (Lichtman, Taylor, Wood, Bluming, & Leibowitz, 1984; Oktay & Walter, 1991; Wellisch, 1981).

Most studies about the consequences of breast cancer focused on individual family member's adjustment, on dyadic family member relationships, and on the family (Irvine, 1996; Lewis & Hammond, 1992; Northouse et al., 1993; Pederson & Valanis, 1988). Prospective studies subsequently examined family functioning and its relationship to family member adjustment when women had breast cancer (Lewis & Hammond, 1992; Lewis, Hammond, & Woods, 1993). Unfortunately, there were far fewer studies about consequences for the family system when the father was diagnosed with cancer and there were children at home.

Qualitative research studies, for example, indicate that women with breast cancer and their families want to be able to move beyond the crisis of the diagnosis and try to maintain normalcy (Buchbinder et al., 2009; Issel et al., 1990). The same would be true for women diagnosed with other types of cancer (Fitch et al., 2000). Fathers diagnosed with cancer also face life plans being challenged as well as possible disruption to their parenting role due to their health status (Buchbinder et al., 2009; O'Neill, McCaughan, Semple, & Ryan, 2013). When faced with a life-threatening illness such as cancer, it may affect a father's ability to be available emotionally and physically to his children as well as being able to provide economically for the family (O'Neill et al., 2013; Torp, Thoresen, Grønningsæter, Grov, & Gustavsen, 2013). Healthcare professionals, therefore, need to be sensitive to and acknowledge the diversity within and between genders and patients' parental roles in order to provide support.

More recently, multinational studies on family functioning as a factor that influences outcomes at the individual and family level when a parent is diagnosed with cancer have been published (Schmitt, Piha, et al., 2008; Thastum et al., 2009). One study involved six European countries (Austria, Denmark, Finland, Germany, Switzerland, and the United Kingdom), a sample of 381 families with 639 parents and 489 children (Schmitt, Piha, Helenius et al., 2008). They continue to be mostly cross-sectional, and this is likely because it is hard to retain families in longitudinal studies and they are more costly to conduct. Despite these limitations, the results from these studies are interesting as there are patterns emerging in the data that remain helpful to healthcare professionals in terms of being able to identify families at risk of poorer health outcomes. The best predictor of internalizing problems in children and adolescents was parental depression, especially in a mother. The best predictor of externalizing problems in children and adolescents was family dysfunction. Therefore, a family-oriented and patient- and family-centered approach is recommended to address the needs of the patient and family.

The Children's and Adolescents' Experience with Cancer in a Parent

Children depend on their parents as their primary source of support. Most of the literature on the experience of cancer among children and adolescents was in the context of a mother's breast cancer (Ellis, Wakefield, Antill, Burns, & Patterson, 2017). Issel et al. (1990) interviewed 81 children, 6–20 years old, of mothers diagnosed with stage I or stage II breast cancer. These authors found keeping family activities as normal, spending time together, and keeping lines of communication open as ways that children perceived their families as helping them to cope. Sadly, more than one third of children reported that their family did nothing to help them to cope. This seemed to be more of a problem for the younger than the older children because more of the older children turned to other adults and friends outside the family for support. Conversely, adolescents' distress might be attributed to feeling pulled to providing support to their mothers at a time when developmentally they need to separate from their family of origin to achieve autonomy (Hilton & Elfert, 1996; Oktay & Walter, 1991; Preto, 1989; Wellisch, 1981). This transition to independence is particularly challenging for adolescent daughters (Compas et al., 1994; Lichtman et al., 1984). If a parent is depressed, then it is even more difficult for their children because the parent may be less accessible for support.

A recent systematic review (Ellis et al., 2017) concluded that children's and adolescents' psychosocial needs when facing cancer in a parent included age-appropriate information about their parent's cancer diagnosis, support in communicating with their parents and other family members, peer support to reduce feelings of isolation and to feel "normal," a safe space to share feelings, individually tailored support to cope with the distress, and specialized support and continued connections, when the parent's cancer progresses and if their parent dies. In addition to exploring challenges for children and adolescents when a parent is diagnosed with cancer, another review also explored challenges related to family functioning and parenting across phases of the illness trajectory to be able to identify appropriate assessment and interventions needs of these families (Kühne et al., 2013).

Parent with Cancer and Children and Adolescents' Reactions

Parent and children's reactions to cancer in a family member have been explored. Studies have examined reactions at time of diagnosis and treatment (Barnes et al., 2000) as well as when there is advanced disease (Kennedy & Lloyd-Williams, 2009; Phillips & Lewis, 2015) or parent in the terminal phase of illness (Buchbinder et al., 2009). Some of the same issues related to communication continue with advanced disease in that parents and their children might want open communication but at the same time try to protect each other (Phillips & Lewis, 2015). Parents have noted that their children and adolescents were resilient. This is based primarily from qualitative studies (Phillips & Lewis, 2015) and less on longitudinal research, which found that the type of communication between parents and their children remained stable over time (Gazendam-Donofrio et al., 2009). Researchers in England (Barnes et al., 2000) identified that mothers with breast cancer would have liked information about how to break news of their diagnosis to their children based upon knowledge of child development. The mothers in their study felt that a meeting as parents, or as a whole family, with a health professional, preferably in their own home would have been helpful, especially thinking that their children might have benefited from talking to a health professional.

Relationship Between Family Functioning and Parents' and Children's Responses

A study conducted in the Netherlands highlighted the multiple factors that can contribute to the response in adolescents 1–5 years after a mother's cancer diagnosis (Huizinga, Visser, Van der Graaf, Hoekstra, Stewart, & Hoekstra-Weebers, 2011). The study reported that 70–80% of 271 adolescents were doing well following the diagnosis and treatment of the mother, whereas 20% of sons and 30% of daughters had an elevated stress response as well as internalizing and externalizing problems. These mental health problems were associated with characteristics of the adolescent (female and older age), parents (more stress response, higher trait anxiety, marital dissatisfaction, and poorer parent-adolescent communication), and illness (intensive treatment and recurrent disease). In fact, the researchers did not find that the time since diagnosis played an important role in adolescent functioning.

Examining the relationship between family functioning and stress responses and psychological functioning in adolescents, researchers in the United Kingdom identified that poor family functioning was an important predictor of adolescents with internalizing problems if the mother had breast cancer (Edwards et al., 2008). The same study identified that poor family cohesion was associated with externalizing problems and increased stress response in these adolescents. Researchers did not find that time since the mother's diagnosis, being on or off chemotherapy, and child's birth order were associated with stress responses. Maternal depression was linked to adolescent-reported internalizing problems. These studies indicate that having a mother with depressive symptoms and families lacking cohesion are potential risk factors for adolescents having psychological problems, likely because of an inability to be attentive to the adolescent's needs. Researcher in Finland found that healthy family functioning such as open communication, flexible problem-solving and appropriate affective involvement predicted less psychological distress in adolescents with a parent with cancer (Lindqvist, Schmitt, Santalahti, Romer, & Piha, 2007).

Screening and Assessment

Likelihood that Patient with Cancer Has Children at Home

The incidence of cancer in parents of minor children (less than 18 years old) is difficult to estimate since tumor registries do not systematically collect demographic statistics about whether a person, who is diagnosed with cancer, has dependent children at home. Most of the information is based upon estimates given age at diagnosis of the patient and likelihood of having children at home. According to Cohn (2013), women as well as men have taken longer to complete their education, establish careers, achieve financial independence from their parents, and get married. Improved birth control methods have enabled women to postpone motherhood. For several decades, the age of first birth among women has increased steadily, so women on average are having their first child later (Mathews & Hamilton, 2016). In the United States and many other nations, it's no longer unusual for women to have a first child at age 35 or even 40 (Cohn, 2013). In Canada, birth rates are higher for women in their late 30s than in their early 20s (Cohn, 2013). The 2016 Canadian census also reported that on average, 34.7% of young Canadians between 20 and 34 years old were living at home with their parents (Statistics Canada, August, 2017), suggesting that parents are having to provide for their children longer into adulthood. This means that if diagnosed with cancer between age 25 and 59 years old, patients are likely to have dependent children at home.

The few studies providing population-based estimates about cancer in a parent were from the United States (Rauch & Moore, 2010; Weaver, Rowland, Alfano, & McNeel, 2010) and Norway (Syse, Aas, & Loge, 2012). In 2003 (Rauch et al.), the National Cancer Institute estimated that 24% of adults with cancer were parenting children under the age of 18. A few years later (Weaver et al., 2010), a US population-based estimate reported that 18% of cancer patients diagnosed in the past 2 years, and 14% of all cancer survivors, were parenting minor children. Semple and McCaugan (2013) reported that up to a third of breast cancer patients were estimated to be parents of minor children in the United Kingdom. In 2007, 3.1% of Norwegian children under the age of 18 had one or both parents with a history of cancer, and the corresponding percentage for young adults was 8.4% (Syse et al., 2012). Therefore, the likelihood that a patient has children at home is dependent upon personal decisions they made about child-rearing and family functioning rather than their cancer diagnosis.

Considering the implications of the finding about the impact of a parent's cancer diagnosis on the family system, it would be important that clinicians ask cancer patients whether there are children still living at home and conduct a more detailed assessment of the family system, including what the children have been told about the parent's cancer and their response. Two family system tools, the genogram and the ecomap, can be used to gather information about the family system and their network of support during a patient or family interview (Friedman et al., 2003; Rolland, 2005). The Distress Thermometer and Canadian Problem Checklist have also been useful tools for screening patient's distress and the problems or concerns that might be contributing to distress (Bultz, Groff, Fitch, et al., 2011; Cancer Journey Portfolio, 2012). Researchers have also developed a questionnaire (PCQ) to assess parenting concerns among adults with cancer (Muriel et al., 2012). The PCQ focuses on the practical impact of the illness on the child, the emotional impact of the illness on the child, and concerns about the co-parent so that a level of parenting distress can be determined. Once having assessed the patient and family, and setting common goals, different intervention strategies can be considered depending upon the concern and whether it is oriented at the patient or family or another family subsystem level.

Interventions Designed to Assist the Ill Parent and Their Family Members

Given the findings of past research, interventions have been designed to improve communication and affective responsiveness, which are components of family functioning thought to be important to assisting the family at multiple levels. This will be explored along with implications for education, appropriate clinical practice, and future research.

Information Resource

Parents diagnosed with cancer and their partners feel that they lack information about how to talk to their children about their diagnosis, and this increases their distress (Barnes et al., 2000; Turner, Yates, Hargraves, & Hausmann, 2007). This was especially true if diagnosed with advanced cancer; therefore, in-depth interviews were conducted with eight Australian women with advanced breast cancer to identify their needs for a brief resource and desired content (Turner et al., 2007). A patient information booklet was created that grouped together information requested such as how to explain advanced cancer and prognosis to children.

Psychosocial Educational Interventions

Parents are considered to be important gatekeepers to children being informed about cancer, and children seemed to have access to variable information about cancer. Therefore, it was thought that having a neutral environment for children to learn about cancer might encourage more open disclosure and learning. Kids Can Cope, an after-school program for children (5–18 years old) whose parents were diagnosed with cancer, was developed in Canada (Taylor-Brown, Acheson, & Farber,

1993). Their parents attended one evening information session, while the children attended six education-based and therapeutic activities. Both benefitted by learning about cancer and children's responses; the children experienced a sense of belonging and learned about the "normal" nature of their feelings and ways of coping.

Another program, known as CLIMB®, was run as a 1.5-h group intervention for children 5–12 years old, run over 6 consecutive weeks by family support workers. It was developed in the United States and adapted in the United Kingdom by Cancer Focus, for children whose parents had cancer (Semple & McCaugan, 2013). Children got together, used art, and play activities to learn basic information about cancer and how to express their emotions. Results indicated that children learned to express and understand their feelings related to having a parent with cancer. Interacting with other children like them led to learning about the experience of other families and normalized their own experience. Feedback from parents was that the children learned more adaptive coping strategies. Some parents wanted concurrent educational sessions to explore communication within the family, children's responses, maintaining routine, and reinforcing parenting responsibilities. Finally, they also recommended that a light dinner be served since the groups occurred in the evening between 5:30 and 7:00 pm, which also interfered with mealtime and homework. So having this would decrease some of their burden as parents.

Kobayashi, Heiney, Osawa, Ozaw, and Matsushima (2017) actually implemented the CLIMB® program with school-aged children and their parents with cancer in Tokyo, Japan. Parents were in separate closed group sessions from their children, which permitted more comfort with disclosure about their experience with cancer. The majority of the parents were mothers with breast cancer. Parents were encouraged to have conversations with their children about their arts and crafts sessions. In the parents' groups, they spoke about their child's emotional state at home or school and family experiences. Results indicated that parents wanted to learn how to talk about cancer-related issues with children and talk to school personnel. Post-traumatic stress scores declined significantly for the children after the intervention compared to before but remained high. Being a single parent and having high post-traumatic stress scores at baseline were thought to be related to a child's stress. The parents' distress scores did not decrease suggesting they were able to deal with parenting concerns related to their children but not their personal suffering.

Strengthening Support Networks

Previous research identified that having a social support network generally had a positive influence on the physical and psychological health of families in crisis. Members of such support networks can feel insecure about how to help families when a parent is diagnosed with cancer (Hauken, Senneseth, Dyrogrov, & Dyregrov, 2015). Therefore, a Norwegian study was developed to evaluate a psychoeducational intervention program for the family and their network of support members. The session lasted about 3 h and could be delivered by a psychologist in the home or other preferred place. The family could choose who they wanted to be involved, and the sessions covered information about cancer, consequences of living with cancer for the ill and healthy parent, children's responses, general reactions and needs of both children and adults, common useful coping strategies, importance of social network of support, importance of openness and communication between family and network, what social networks can do, and types of support as well as how to sustain them. Partners facing spousal cancer reported more psychological distress and lower quality of life than other healthy Norwegians (Senneseth, Hauken, Matthieeson, Gjestad, & Laberg, 2017).

Families that receive help from their network of support members potentially report a feeling of reduced burden, which consequently allows for more time for self-care (Hauken et al., 2015). The clinical implication for healthcare professionals is that they need to pay attention not only to the mental health of the ill parent but also their parenting partner. Together with talking about how they are managing the care for their children and about their need for support, healthcare professionals may be able to help parents mobilize their social network for instrumental and emotional support.

Educational and School-Based Interventions

Parents might want teachers to monitor their children for changes in school performance and behavior and to provide support, but parents did not always know how to seek such support (Fasciano et al., 2007; Rossy Cancer Network, 2017). To be able to support children and parents challenged by a cancer diagnosis and treatment, school-based personnel wanted information regarding impact of cancer on families and effective ways of supporting families dealing with parental cancer, including communication with child and family (Fasciano et al., 2007). Therefore, Fasciano et al. (2007) and colleagues conducted an evaluation of a community-based program for school personnel modeled on one developed by *The Wellness Community* in the United States for people with cancer and their loved ones. The results indicated school-based personnel felt significantly more knowledgeable and equipped with effective ways of supporting children and families dealing with parental cancer. School-based personnel learned to reach out and listen to families' needs. Prior personal experience with cancer and school-based personnel having supported several families facing cancer contributed to less anxiety dealing with children and families.

Talking to a child or teen about a parent's cancer has to be one of the toughest things a caregiver ever has to face. But not talking about it can be even worse as it can cause anxiety and distress for the children as well as their parents. In 2013, the Canadian Association of Psychosocial Oncology (www.capo.ca) developed a web-based educational program for healthcare providers and school-based personnel to be able to support children and adolescents when someone close to them had cancer. With the help of the Rossy Cancer Network (Rossy Cancer Network, 2017), the web-based modules were adapted for patients in an English and a French version (www.startthetalk.ca; www.parlonsen.ca). "Children pick up cues, they're aware something is going on but they're not quite sure what...The older ones can figure it out but the younger ones can't and, especially in families where some people know and others don't, it leads to a lot of anxiety" (Rossy Cancer Network, 2017, p. 7). The quality of care improvement project had as objectives to provide healthcare providers, school-based personnel, cancer patients, and their families the tools to address cancer with children and teens who are affected by the illness, as well as to increase accessibility and awareness. "We want to empower patients to be able to open up the discussion with their care team and develop some comfort in bringing up the topic with children and teens," explained Dr. Laizner (Rossy Cancer Network, 2017, p. 7). The interactive website uses videos, slides, images, text, and testimonials to convey in simple terms what cancer is, what children understand at different ages, ways to help them cope, and tips on how to discuss the stages of the disease, including diagnosis, treatment, recurrence, and death. There is also a list of other resources, including age-appropriate books and other online materials for children and adolescents, parents, and health professionals within each module.

A survey of 131 ambulatory cancer patients and 88 healthcare providers in April 2016 revealed that a very small proportion – 4% – of patients and 16% of healthcare professionals were aware of the [existing CAPO] modules (Rossy Cancer Network, 2017, p. 7). To turn this around, multipronged dissemination strategies have been implemented (oral presentations mostly to nurses and patients, e-blasts, and bookmarks with web address of the resource) by project team members. In 2016, website visits almost doubled during the period of the information sessions. A follow-up survey will be done toward the end of 2017 (Rossy Cancer Network, 2017). Therefore, when creating e-learning educational materials, it is important to monitor accessibility, awareness, use, and usefulness of the materials for their target population.

Summary and Discussion

This chapter has highlighted some of the important consequences reported by family members about their needs and family functioning. Based upon demographic information and previous research results, innovative interventions have been explored based upon a family systems perspective (Ellis et al., 2017). They were developed to respond to the psychosocial needs of family members when a parent has been diagnosed with cancer and selected examples have been presented in an attempt to inform clinical programs and services.

Implications for Clinical Practice and Future Research

The development of parent- and family-centered competent care for parents with cancer and their minor children should be a priority for oncology and healthcare providers. Researchers are still questioning how interventions should be targeted (Lewis, 2004, 2007). It is important for clinicians to respond appropriately to the specific needs of parents with cancer and their family members. Whether all family members need to be involved is not clear. Research does identify that transparent age-appropriate communication and emotional support needs to be a priority with the children, therefore, parents require education and understanding during all phases of the illness journey including the survivorship experience and bereavement (Ellis et al., 2017).

Healthcare professionals need to help parents remain in control by providing information and guidance while making important decisions about treatment and care needs for themselves and their family. Establishing effective interdisciplinary communication is necessary to address the needs of at-risk family members when a parent is diagnosed with cancer. Survivorship issues continue to exist as well as cancer treatments improve, and it is seen as a chronic illness with risk of recurrence and issues related to loss and bereavement if a parent is diagnosed with advanced cancer.

Future research and policy interventions should focus on enhancing community supports by providing support in schools as well as appropriate health services that are patient and family centered. Young children and adolescents should be directed toward peer support activities and services that address their needs and promote their own development. Additionally, and of equal importance, future investigations are needed to evaluate the education and training of oncology and healthcare professionals focusing not only on the disease and medical treatment but on the psychosocial needs of a parent with cancer and their family. School-based professionals, healthcare workers, and oncology professionals should remain open to new knowledge, differing beliefs about family functioning, and innovative ways to provide information and support, which hopefully will better serve these families.

References

Anderson, S. A., & Sabatelli, R. M. (2011). *Family interaction: A multigenerational developmental perspective* (5th ed.). Boston, MA: Allyn & Bacon.

Barnes, J., Kroll, L., Burke, O., Lee, J., Jones, A., & Stein, A. (2000). Qualitative interview study of communication between parents and their children about maternal breast cancer. *British Medical Journal, 321*, 479–482.

Buchbinder, M. A., Longhofer, J., & McCue, K. (2009). Family routines and rituals when a parent has cancer. *Families, Systems, & Health, 27*, 213–227.

Bultz, B. D., Groff, S. L., Fitch, M., et al. (2011). Implementing screening for distress, the 6th vital sign: A Canadian strategy for changing practice. *Psycho-Oncology, 20*, 463–469.

Cancer Journey Portfolio. (2012). Screening for distress, the 6th vital sign: A guide to implementing best practice in person-centered care. www.cancerview.ca

Cohn, D. V. (2013, 10 July). In Canada most babies now born to women 30 and older. PEW Research Center, July 10, 2013. Washington, DC. http://www.pewresearch.org/fact-tank/2013/07/10/in-canada-most-babies-now-born-to-women-30-and-older/

Compas, B. E., Worsham, N. L., Epping-Jordan, J. E., Grant, K. E., Mireault, G., Howell, D. C., & Malcarne, V. L. (1994). When mom or dad has cancer: Markers of psychological distress in cancer patients, spouses, and children. *Health Psychology, 13*, 507–515.

Edwards, L., Watson, M., St. James-Roberts, I., Ashley, S., Tilney, C., Brougham, B., … Romer, G. (2008). Adolescent's stress responses and the psychological functioning when a parent has early breast cancer. *Psycho-Oncology, 17*, 1039–1047.

Ellis, S. J., Wakefield, C. E., Antill, G., Burns, M., & Patterson, P. (2017). Supporting children facing a parent's cancer diagnosis: A systematic review of children's psychosocial needs and existing interventions. *European Journal of Cancer Care, 26*, e12432. https://doi.org/10.1111/ecc.12432

Fasciano, K. M., Berman, H., Moore, C., DeFrino, B., Jameson, R., Kennedy, V., & Golant, M. (2007). When a parent has cancer: A community based program for school personnel. *Psycho-Oncology, 16*, 158–167.

Fitch, M., Gray, R. E., & Franssen, E. (2000). Perspectives on living with ovarian cancer: Young women's views. *Canadian Oncology Nursing Journal, 10*(3), 101–108.

Friedman, L. C., Baer, P. E., Nelson, D. V., Lane, M., Smith, F. E., & Dworkin, R. J. (1988). Women with breast cancer: Perception of family functioning and adjustment to illness. *Psychosomatic Medicine, 50*, 529–540.

Friedman, M. M., Bowden, V. R., & Jones, E. G. (2003). *Family nursing: Research, theory, and practice* (5th ed.). Upper Saddle River, NJ: Prentice Hall.

Gazendam-Donofrio, S., Hoekstra, H., van der Graaf, W., van der Wiel, H., Visser, A., Huizinga, G., & Hoekstra-Weebers, J. (2009). Parent-child communication patterns during first year after a parent's cancer diagnosis: The effect on parent functioning. *Cancer, 115*, 4227–4237.

Grabiak, B. R., Bender, C. M., & Puskar, K. R. (2007). The impact of parental cancer on the adolescent: An analysis of the literature. *Psycho-Oncology, 16*, 127–137.

Hauken, M. A., Senneseth, M., Dyrogrov, A., & Dyregrov, K. (2015). Optimizing social network support to families living with parental cancer: Research protocol for the Cancer PEPSONE Study. *JIMR Research Protocols, 4*(4), e142. https://doi.org/10.2196/resprot.4055

Hilton, B. A. (1993a). Issues, problems, and challenges for families coping with breast cancer. *Seminars in Oncology Nursing, 9*, 88–100.

Hilton, B. A. (1993b). A study of couple communication patterns when coping with early stage breast cancer. *Canadian Oncology Nursing Journal, 3*(4), 159–166.

Hilton, B. A. (1994). Family communication patterns in coping with early breast cancer. *Western Journal in Nursing Research, 16*, 366–391.

Hilton, B. A., & Elfert, H. (1996). Children's experiences with mothers' early breast cancer. *Cancer Practice, 4*, 96–104.

Hilton, B. A., & Gustavason, K. (2002). Shielding and being shielded: Children's perspectives on coping with their mother's cancer and chemotherapy. *Canadian Oncology Nursing Journal, 12*(4), 198–206.

Huizinga, G. A., Visser, A., Van der Graaf, W. T. A., Hoekstra, H. J., Stewart, R. E., & Hoekstra-Weebers, J. E. H. M. (2011). Family-oriented multilevel study on the psychological functioning of adolescents children having a mother with cancer. *Psycho-Oncology, 20*, 730–737.

Irvine, D. M. (1996). *A critical review and meta-analysis of the literature investigating psychosocial adjustment in breast cancer*. Ottawa, ON: Health Canada, Minister of Supply and Services Canada.

Issel, L. M., Ersek, M., & Lewis, F. M. (1990). How children cope with mother's breast cancer. *Oncology Nursing Forum, 17*, 5–12.

Kennedy, V. L., & Lloyd-Williams, M. (2009). How children cope when a parent has advanced cancer. *Psycho-Oncology, 18*, 886–892.

Kobayashi, M., Heiney, S. P., Osawa, K., Ozaw, M., & Matsushima, E. (2017). Effect of a group intervention for children and their parents who have cancer. *Palliative and Supportive Care*. https://doi.org/10.1017/S1478951516001115

Krauel, K., Simon, A., Krause-Hebecker, N., Czimbalmos, A., Bottomley, A., & Flechtner, H. (2012). When a parent has cancer: Challenges to patients, their families and health providers. *Expert Reviews Pharmacoecon: Outcomes Research, 12*, 795–808.

Kühne, F., Krattenmacher, T., Bergelt, C., Beierlein, V., Herzog, W. V., Klitzing, K., … Möller, B. (2013). There is still so much ahead of us – Family functioning in families of palliative cancer patients. *Families, Systems, & Health, 31*, 181–193.

Lewis, F. M. (2004). Family-focused oncology nursing research. *Oncology Nursing Forum, 31*, 288–292.

Lewis, F. M. (2007). Parental cancer and dependent children: Selected issues for future research. *Psycho-Oncology, 16*, 97–98.
Lewis, F. M., & Hammond, M. A. (1992). Psychosocial adjustment of the family to breast cancer: A longitudinal analysis. *Journal of the American Medical Women's Association, 47*, 194–200.
Lewis, F. M., Hammond, M. A., & Woods, N. F. (1993). The family's functioning with newly diagnosed breast cancer in the mother: The development of an explanatory model. *Journal of Behavioral Medicine, 16*, 351–370.
Lewis, F. M., Woods, N. F., Hough, E. E., & Bensley, L. S. (1989). The family's functioning with chronic illness in the mother: The spouse's perspective. *Social Science & Medicine, 29*, 1261–1269.
Lewis, F. M., Zahlis, E. H., Shands, M. E., Sinsheimer, J. A., & Hammond, M. A. (1996). The functioning of single women with breast cancer and their school-aged children. *Cancer Practice, 4*, 15–24.
Lichtman, R. R., Taylor, S. E., Wood, J. V., Bluming, A. Z., Dosik, G. M., & Leibowitz, R. L. (1984). Relations with children after breast cancer. The mother-daughter relationship at risk. *Journal of Psychosocial Oncology, 2*(3/4), 1–19.
Lindqvist, B., Schmitt, F., Santalahti, P., Romer, G., & Piha, J. (2007). Factors associated with the mental health of adolescents when a parent has cancer. *Scandinavian Journal of Psychology, 48*, 345–351.
Maguire, P. (1981). Repercussions of mastectomy on the family. *International Journal of Family Psychiatry, 1*, 485–503.
Mathews, T. J., & Hamilton, B. E. (2016, January). Mean age of mothers is on the rise: United States, 2000–2014 *NCHS Data Brief, No. 232*. Hyattsville, MD: National Center for Health Statistics. 2016. www.cdc.gov/nchs/data/databriefs/db232.pdf
Muriel, A. C., Moore, C. W., Baer, L., Park, E. R., Kornnblith, A. B., Pirl, W., … Rauch, P. K. (2012). Measuring psychosocial distress and parenting concerns among adults with cancer. *Cancer, 118*, 5671–5678.
Northouse, L. (1990). A longitudinal study of the adjustment of patients and husbands to breast cancer. *Oncology Nursing Forum, 17*((3 Suppl.)), 39–45.
Northouse, L. L., Cracchiolo-Caraway, A., & Appel, C. P. (1993). Psychologic consequences of breast cancer on partner and family. *Seminars in Oncology Nursing, 7*, 216–223.
Northouse, L. L., & Swain, M. A. (1987). Adjustment of patients and husbands to the initial impact of breast cancer. *Nursing Research, 36*, 221–225.
O'Neill, C., McCaughan, E., Semple, C., & Ryan, A. (2013). Fatherhood and cancer: A commentary on the literature. *European Journal of Cancer Care, 22*, 161–168.
Oktay, J. S., & Walter, C. A. (1991). *Breast cancer in the life course*. New York, NY: Springer.
Osborn, T. (2007). The psychosocial impact of parental cancer on children and adolescents: A systematic review. *Psycho-Oncology, 16*, 101–126.
Pederson, L. M., & Valanis, B. G. (1988). The effects of breast cancer on the family: A review of the literature. *Journal of Psychosocial Oncology, 6*, 95–118.
Phillips, F. (2014). Adolescent living with a parent with advanced cancer: A review of the literature. *Psycho-Oncology, 23*, 1323–1339.
Phillips, F., & Lewis, F. M. (2015). The adolescent's experience when a parent has advanced cancer: A qualitative inquiry. *Palliative Medicine, 29*, 851–858.
Preto, N. G. (1989). Transformation of the family system in adolescence. In B. Carter & M. McGoldrick (Eds.), *The changing family life cycle* (pp. 255–283). Boston, MA: Allyn & Bacon.
Purc-Stephensen, R., & Lyseng, A. (2016). How are the kids holding up? A systematic review and meta-analysis on the psychosocial impact of maternal breast cancer on children. *Cancer Treatment Reviews, 49*, 45–56.
Rauch, P., & Moore, C. (2010). A population-based estimate of cancer survivors residing with minor children. *Cancer, 116*, Editorial, September 15. https://doi.org/10.1002/cncr.25360
Rolland, J. (2005). Cancer and the family: An integrative model. *Cancer, 104*(11 Suppl), 2584–2595.

Rossy Cancer Network (2017, Summer). Innovation: Spreading the word. RCN Update, Montreal, QC: Rossy Cancer Network, p. 7. http://mcgill.ca/rcr-rcn/files/rcr-rcn/rcn_newsletter_summer_2017.pdf.

Schmitt, F., Piha, J., Helenius, H., Baldus, C., Kienbacher, C., Steck, B., … Romer, G. (2008). Multinational study of cancer patients and their children: Factors associated with family functioning. *Journal of Clinical Oncology*, *26*, 5877–5883.

Semple, C. J., & McCaugan, E. (2013). Family life when a parent is diagnosed with cancer: Impact of a psychosocial intervention for young children. *European Journal of Cancer Care*, *22*, 219–231.

Senneseth, M., Hauken, M. A., Matthieeson, S. B., Gjestad, R., & Laberg, J. C. (2017). Facing spousal cancer during child-rearing years. *Cancer Nursing*, *40*(3), E24–E34.

Statistics Canada (2017, August). Census of population, 2016. Census in brief: Young adults living with their parents in Canada in 2016. http://www12.statcan.gc.ca/census-recensement/2016/as-sa/98-200-x/2016008/98-200-x2016008-eng.cfm.

Syse, A., Aas, G. B., & Loge, J. H. (2012). Children and young adults with parents with cancer: A population-based study. *Clinical Epidemiology*, *4*, 41–52.

Taylor-Brown, J., Acheson, A., & Farber, J. (1993). Kids can cope: A group intervention for children whose parents have cancer. *Journal of Psychosocial Oncology*, *11*, 41–53.

Thastum, M., Watson, M., Kienbacher, C., Piha, J., Steck, B., Zachariae, R., … Romer, G. (2009). Prevalence and predictors of emotional and behavioural functioning of children where a parent has cancer: A multinational study. *Cancer*, *115*, 4030–4039.

Torp, S., Thoresen, L., Grønningsæter, A. B., Grov, E. K., & Gustavsen, K. (2013). Financial and social effects on children and adolescents when a parent is diagnosed with cancer. *Child Adolescent Social Work*, *30*, 293–310.

Turner, J., Yates, P., Hargraves, M., & Hausmann, S. (2007). Development of a resource for parents with advanced cancer: What do parents want? *Palliative and Supportive Care*, *5*, 135–145.

Walsh, F. (2012). *Normal family processes: Growing diversity and complexity* (4th ed.). New York, NY: Guilford Press.

Weaver, K. E., Rowland, J. H., Alfano, C. M., & McNeel, T. S. (2010). Parental cancer and the family: A population-based estimate of the number of US cancer survivors residing with their minor children. *Cancer*, *116*, 4395–4401.

Wellisch, D. K. (1981). Family relationships of the mastectomy patient: Interactions with the spouse and children. *Israel Journal of Medical Sciences*, *17*, 993–996.

Chapter 12
When Cancer Returns: Survivors, Caregivers, and the Family System

Suzanne Young Bushfield

Purpose

The purpose of this chapter is to identify the needs of cancer survivors and their caregivers when cancer returns and to describe family systems theory as an organizing framework for appropriate interventions to improve care for cancer survivors and their caregivers through end-of-life care.

Introduction

Surviving cancer is increasingly more common, due in part to improved rates and methods for early detection and newer treatment modalities. Long-term effects of cancer have therefore received more attention, as survivorship (defined as surviving cancer diagnosis by 5 years or more) is often accompanied by patient concerns such as fatigue, pain, fear of recurrence, depression, and isolation. In addition, caregivers and family members report psychosocial concerns that are similar to patients. Interventions for survivors and caregivers have focused on social support and education, as well as methods for reducing anxiety and fear of recurrence. Nevertheless, when cancer returns as metastatic and advanced disease, patients with cancer and their caregivers must adapt to new uncertainties and cope with the reality of end-of-life decisions. As with other crises, a cancer diagnosis has an impact on the entire family system. A family system perspective provides a useful framework for understanding the family as the unit of care, across the trajectory of cancer survivorship and particularly when cancer returns (Bushfield & DeFord, 2010).

S. Y. Bushfield (✉)
Suzanne Young Bushfield, School of Social Work, Arizona State University, Tempe, AZ, USA

T. R. Fitzpatrick (ed.), *Quality of Life Among Cancer Survivors*,
https://doi.org/10.1007/978-3-319-75223-5_12

Literature Review

Survivorship

With nearly 14 million cancer survivors in the United States, women make up 54% of cancer survivors (National Cancer Institute, 2012). Survivors of cancer have benefitted from two key factors: early detection and improved treatment (CDC, 2015). Early detection is known to significantly reduce mortality (Cedolini, Bertozzi, Londero, & Bernardi, 2014; Grabler, Dupuy, Raj, Bernstein, & Ansell, 2012). As cancer death rates continue to decline, attention to survivorship concerns has grown. Survivors of cancer often experience a number of health challenges, including pain, fatigue, cognitive changes, weight loss or gain, sexual dysfunction, as well as fear of recurrence (National Cancer Institute, 2014). This fear is not unfounded: even though early detection and effective treatments have improved survivorship, the risk of relapse or recurrence persists even 15 years after initial diagnosis (Natarajan et al., 2009). Both caregivers and survivors have identified lasting life changes following diagnosis and treatment from cancer. Positive changes (such as a change in perspective or a different outlook on life) and negative changes (such as lingering health effects) are both long lasting (Bishop, Curbow, Springert, Lee, & Wingard, 2011). Other issues have been found to have a significant impact on survivorship, notably economic burden and fear of reoccurrence (American Cancer Society, 2015). Geographic inequalities due to remoteness and socioeconomic disadvantage have been identified (Dasgupta, 2012). For women in rural communities or without proximity to regional cancer centers, disparities may be magnified (Peek & Han, 2004). The timeliness of follow-up care is also important. Longer intervals between initial diagnosis and treatment result in poorer outcomes (Olivetto, Gomi, & Bancej, 2002; Jones, Dailey, & Calvocoressi, 2005), and women in rural areas, those with lower incomes, and minorities are among those with long intervals between diagnosis and treatment.

The shift from understanding cancer as an acute illness to recognizing it as a chronic disease, with long-term consequences that may be both positive and negative, represents a paradigm shift in health care (Hebdon, Foli, & McComb, 2015). The transition from patient to survivor is also a challenge to patients and their caregivers (Mollica, & Nemeth, 2015; Taplin et al., 2010). Some do not wish to identify themselves as survivors and reject the term "survivor" (Hebdon et al., 2015). Nevertheless, they acknowledge the importance of support in a variety of ways, not limited to traditional support groups (Morris et al., 2014). While a focus on survivorship may have increased appropriate interventions across the trajectory of cancer care, survivors and their caregivers face new challenges when cancer returns.

Fear and Relapse

Adapting to, and surviving from, cancer may be a lifelong process of reappraisal and adjustment over time (Naus, Ishler, Parrott, & Kovacs, 2009). Due to the long trajectory of cancer survivorship for some, fear of recurrence may be both a long-term and realistic concern. The centrality of cancer survivorship in one's self concept has been linked to engaging in behaviors to support well-being and with greater psychological distress (Helgeson, 2011). The latter was present when the central concept of being a cancer survivor was present and when cancer was viewed in more negative terms. Some 83% of cancer survivors identify themselves as "survivors" as opposed to "patients" or "victims" (Park, Zlateva, & Blank, 2009). Uncertainty during the transition from patient to survivor is very common during active treatment for cancer (Garofalo (2009). When relapse occurs, that uncertainty may increase for both patients and their caregivers. Further, caregivers may be so engrossed in the duties of daily caregiving that they are unable to clearly identify their own needs and fears (Rabow, Hauser, & Adams, 2004). Fear of cancer recurrence is related to poorer quality of life, and greater levels of fear are associated with the severity of the cancer diagnosis in both survivors and their caregivers (Kim, Carver, Spillers, Love-Ghaffari, & Kaw, 2012).

Social Support

Social support has been identified as a strong predictor for a positive prognosis (DeBoer, Ryckman, Pruyn, & Van den Borne, 1999). Social support (both instrumental and emotional) helps buffer the effects of stress (Spiegel, Sephton, Terr, & Stites, 1998). Even though some survivors may reject identification of themselves as "survivors," they acknowledge the importance of receiving support in a variety of ways, not limited to traditional support groups Morris et al. (2014). Some cancer survivors may be more sensitive to social support (Declerck, DeBrabander, Boone, & Gerits, 2002). Caregiver support may have an even longer trajectory (Bushfield, 2016); support for caregivers, when provided early, may yield protection against negative outcomes into bereavement (Gustavson & Dal Santo, 2008).

Family Caregiving and Caregiver Needs

The stress of family caregiving can be overwhelming (Hebert, Copeland, Schulz, Amato, & Arnold, 2008). At the end of life, caregivers spend an average of 100 hours a week providing care (Haley et al. 2010, as cited in Morrow & Nicholson, 2016). Some 45 million adults provide long-term, unpaid care to a loved one, and many of those caregivers (nearly 80%) are over age 50 (National Alliance for Caregiving,

2007). Additional challenges occur when the patient/survivor has been the main caregiver within the family, and now others, not used to the caregiver role, must assume those duties and responsibilities.

Caregivers for patients with cancer describe a variety of multidimensional needs, including physical, psychological, social, and spiritual and experienced challenges in all four of those domains (Skalla, Smith, Li, & Gates, 2013). Among these concerns are fatigue, insomnia, and financial issues. Most caregivers reported a baseline level of distress and anxiety at the time of the patient's diagnosis; they also maintained that level of distress across the trajectory of survivorship (Lambert, Jones, Girgis, & Lecathelinais, 2012). Many caregivers have unmet needs for information and emotional support, particularly for their fears (Sklenarova, Krumpelmann, & Haun, 2015). The extent to which caregivers' psychosocial needs were unmet was a strong predictor of poor mental health across the trajectory of survivorship, pointing to a need for interventions that can be useful across the trajectory of care (Kim, Kashy, Spillers, & Eans, 2010). This need is very evident at the end of life. Caregivers for a loved one who is dying have increased burden and report that they feel unprepared for the end of life (Hebert et al., 2008; Teno et al., 2004, Barry & Prigerson, 2002). This lack of preparation for death, including information, support, and effective communication from health-care providers, leads to additional complications for the caregivers that extend into bereavement (Barry et al., 2006; Hebert, Dang, & Schulz, 2006; Hebert et al., 2008). Further, cancer and its recurrence may generate spiritual and existential concerns for both survivors and caregivers.

Family Systems

Family systems theory, developed by Murray Bowen (Kerr & Bowen, 1988), is a theory that attempts to explain the multidimensional complexities of relationships, behaviors, and feelings within the family unit and between family members and the outside world. As originally conceived, family systems theory views the family as an emotional unit. The complex interactions within the family unit are best understood by recognizing that the entire unit is impacted by a change in any of its parts; the system must struggle to adapt to those changes. Illness, survivorship, caregiving, and death are not, therefore, individual experiences, but rather transitions; their accompanying losses are experienced by each member of the family unit. From this perspective, formal and informal caregivers, including medical professionals, psychosocial and spiritual caregivers, and others involved in care and treatment, become part of the larger system of care that is interacting with and experiencing the loss associated with cancer recurrence (Bushfield & DeFord, 2010).

Families begin as our primary relationships. What we learn about how to relate, how to get along, how to be together, and how to separate is first developed from within our family system (Bushfield & DeFord, 2010). The struggles of the family system to accommodate change are impacted by many variables.

Bowen described two primary variables in family systems. First is the *differentiation of self*. The competing needs of separating, or being an autonomous individual, and the need to be connected, or a sense of togetherness in relationships, are conflicting forces constantly working within each individual. The balance between these two competing needs is modified by the family system, which exerts a pull toward togetherness. The second variable in the Bowen systems approach is *chronic anxiety*. Bowen describes this as a result of the system's attempt to achieve balance or equilibrium. When family systems are more flexible or less rigid, they are better able to adapt to change without increasing anxiety beyond a manageable level (Bushfield & DeFord, 2010).

Application to Survivorship and Recurrence

For some, cancer recurrence is experienced as a failure: treatment did not work; what was the reason? Adapting to the loss of survivorship and facing death may carry a sense of failure and shame (Bushfield & DeFord, 2010). Mourning becomes the "new normal" as the family system struggles to adapt to physical, psychosocial, and spiritual challenges of illness and the anticipatory grief that comes with a terminal diagnosis.

Survivorship care plans are intended to address the holistic needs and concerns for cancer survivors, such as recognizing emotions, accepting fears, reducing stress, staying well informed, receiving follow-up health care, making healthy choices, and nurturing strong support systems (American Cancer Society, 2015). With a terminal diagnosis, patients and caregivers have additional tasks: adapting hope to new uncertainties and facing death (Bushfield & Deford, 2010).

There is a good reason to include the entire family system in care plans. All of these adaptations are not for the survivor/patient alone; caregivers and the family system are simultaneously adapting to new responsibilities. As the survivor becomes a patient once again, caregiver burden increases. While patients/survivors talk about their experiences as "I," caregivers, reporting similar concerns and experiences, typically describe their experiences and adjustments as "we" (Jo et al., 2007).

Implications for Practice at the End of Life

Relapse fear may be mitigated by providing information to caregivers and their families, but specific interventions focused on decreasing fear have demonstrated positive effects (Montesinos & Luciano, 2016). Rather than thought suppression or avoidance as a coping strategy, exposure may promote greater psychological flexibility (Montesinos & Luciano, 2016). Exposure might also be described as assisting patients in thinking about the fears that they experience, rather than trying to avoid those thoughts. Decreasing the interference of fears may promote more active engagement with others in meaningful interchanges. In a family system approach, regulating the emotional reactivity in the family by reducing anxiety promotes a climate which allows the family system to adapt more readily to the difficult changes that end-of-life care brings (Bushfield & DeFord, 2010).

Caregiving is far from an abstract concept; it is a personal experience of interdependence; it is relational (Bushfield & DeFord, 2010). From that standpoint, how families respond to giving and receiving care reflects how a family system manages anxiety when its homeostasis is in transition. The dependency of the patient demands dependability from the caregivers. Adjustment to this and other changes may create more volatility. Interventions which seek to support the caregiver in their many tasks and communicate more effectively may assist the entire family system in facing death.

Caregivers and patients report that gaining a sense of control increases hope; this sense of control may be enhanced by social support in some cancer survivors (Declerck et al., 2002). When caregivers provide a non-anxious presence, prompting all members of the family system to think about what they are feeling, they can assist in reducing anxiety and improving quality of life, even at the end of life (Bushfield & DeFord).

Holistic care at the end of life includes spiritual care. An individual's religious norms and beliefs are seen as central to one's understanding of illness (Zeilani, 2012). Spiritual well-being is associated with improved mental health and quality of life (Kim, Carver, Spillers, Crammer, & Zhou, 2011). Spiritual well-being and the ability to find meaning and peace at the end of life may contribute to overall well-being for both survivors/patients and their caregivers/family systems (Kim et al., 2011). The importance of assessing the saliency of religion or worldview in one's life is fundamental to addressing the spiritual needs of others (Hodge & Bushfield, 2006, Van Hook et al., 2001). While the need for measures which are more subtle than broad based has been identified (Hodge, 2004; Koenig & Bussing, 2010), competent spiritual assessment should be included in end-of-life care. Spiritual competence, as an aspect of holistic treatment, should be viewed as an active, ongoing process characterized by three ongoing and interrelated dimensions: growing awareness of one's spiritual world view and associated assumptions, limitations, and biases; a developing empathic understanding of other's spiritual worldview that is devoid of judgment; and an increasing ability to design and implement appropriate and relevant interventions that are sensitive to others' world view (Hodge, 2004; Hodge & Bushfield, 2006). This sensitivity is particularly important for families facing end-of-life decision-making (Bushfield & DeFord, 2010). Isolation and loneliness are common in cancer patients and their caregivers Rosedale (2009). This isolation may be a function of awareness of mortality and the existential threat of cancer. The heightened distress experienced by survivors, including survival guilt, may also have a spiritual dimension (Maxwell & Aldredge-Clanton, 1994; Miller & Thoresen, 2003).

Care for caregivers requires a multidimensional assessment. Each survivor/patient and their caregivers/family systems are unique. Understanding the specific context of the caregiver; the caregiver's own perception of the health and functional status of the one receiving care; the caregiver's values, preferences, and worldview; the caregiver's well-being; the caregiver's skills, abilities, and knowledge base for providing care as well as their limitations in these areas; and the potential resources available to the caregiver all serve to support a family system perspective (National Alliance for Family Caregiving, 2007; Bushfield & DeFord, 2010).

Conclusions

Surviving cancer has become the "new normal" for millions of patients. Yet, the transition from patient to survivor is a road that is sometimes difficult to navigate. Survivorship may be improved by the presence of social support, most often provided by family caregivers. These caregivers experience similar challenges, describing the cancer survivor's diagnosis, illness, and treatment experiences as "we" versus the "I" descriptions of the patient (Jo et al., 2007). A family systems approach recognizes that the family unit should be the focus of interventions to address needs for information and social support, as well as needs to address fears of relapse, fatigue, and financial burden. When cancer returns, caregivers bear the burden of keeping hope alive while adapting to new realities. End-of-life interventions need to support the family systems, without judgment, through a non-anxious presence, in order to allow the family system to adjust to new realities. The adaption of the family system to relapse may create new anxieties, as grief and loss escalate. Family caregivers and health-care providers, including hospice team members, must seek to enter the family system for end-of-life care by identifying emotional processes and assisting the family in its adjustment to the trajectory which extends through bereavement care. Being present, but not intrusive, and finding ways to help the family members gain a sense of control even when feelings are out of control can be of great support to families facing death (Beckman, 2016). Supporting the caregiver, encouraging self-care and sleep when possible, and feeling comfortable being with grief can ease some of the unbearable burden at the end of life (Cacciatore, 2017).

References

American Cancer Society (2015). *Survivorship care plans*. Atlanta, GA: American Cancer Society Information Center.

Barry, D. B. (2006). Statistical Issues: Barr et al. Respond. In Environmental Health Perspectives. *National Institute of Environmental Health Services, 114*(12), A689–A690.

Barry, L. C., & Prigerson, H. G. (2002). Perspectives on preparedness for death among bereaved persons. *Conn Med, 66*, 691–696.

Beckman, S. (2016). Alongside: A Practical guide for loving your neighbor in their time of trial. New York, NY: Morgan James Faith.

Bishop, M. M., Curbow, B. A., Springert, S. H., Lee, J. A., & Wingard, J. R. (2011). Comparison of lasting life changes after cancer and bone marrow transplant: Perspectives of long-term survivors and spouses. *Psycho-Oncology, 20*(9), 926–934.

Bushfield, S. (2016). Survivorship issues among Muslim women with cancer, Ch. 4 (pp. 55–65). In T. Fitzpatrick (Ed.), *Treating vulnerable populations of cancer survivors: A biopsychosocial approach*. New York, NY: Springer Co.

Bushfield, S., & DeFord, B. (2010). *End of life care and addiction: A family systems approach*. New York, NY: Springer.

Cacciatore, J. (2017). B*earing the unbearable: Love, loss, and the heartbreaking pain of grief.* Summerville, MA: Wisdom Publications.

Cedolini, C., Bertozzi, S., Londero, A. P., & Bernardi, S. (2014). Type of breast cancer diagnosis, screening, and survival. *Clinical Breast Cancer, 14*(4), 235–240.

Centers for Disease Control (CDC) and Prevention, Cancer Screening. (2012). *Morbidity and Mortality Report, 61*(3), 41–45.

Centers for Disease Control and Prevention (CDC) (2015). *Cancer screening United States*. Atlanta, GA: U.S. Department of Human Services Centers for Disease Control and Prevention and National Cancer Institute.

Dasgupta, P. (2012). Multilevel determinants of breast cancer survival: Association with geographic remoteness and area-level socioeconomic disadvantage. *Breast Cancer Research and Treatment, 132*(2), 701–710.

DeBoer, M. F., Ryckman, R. M., Pruyn, J. F., & Van den Borne, W. H. (1999). Psychosocial correlates of cancer relapse and survival: A literature review. *Patient Education and Counseling, 37*, 215–230.

Declerck, C. H., DeBrabander, B., Boone, C., & Gerits, P. (2002). Locus of control, marital status and predictors of early relapse in primary breast cancer patients. *Psychology and Health, 17*(1), 63–76.

Garofalo, J. (2009). Uncertainty during the transition from cancer patient to survivor. *Cancer Nursing, 32*(4), E8–E14.

Grabler, P., Dupuy, D., Raj, J., Bernstein, S., & Ansell, D. (2012). Regular screening mammography before the diagnosis of breast cancer reduces black/white breast cancer differences and modifies negative prognostic factors. *Breast Cancer Research and Treatment, 135*, 549–553.

Gustavson, K., & Dal Santo, T. (2008). Caregiver service use: A complex story of care at the end of life. *Journal of Social Work in End-of-Life & Palliative Care, 4*(4), 286–311.

Hebdon, M., Foli, K., & McComb, S. (2015). Survivor in the cancer context. *Journal of Advanced Nursing, 71*(8), 1774–1786.

Hebert, R., Copeland, V. C., Schulz, R., Amato, C. A., & Arnold, R. M. (2008). Preparing family caregivers for the death of a loved one: Implications for hospital social workers. *Journal of Social Work & Palliative Care, 4*(4), 269–285.

Hebert, R. S., Dang, Q., & Schulz, R. (2006). Caring for caregivers: the essence of palliative care. *Journal of Palliative Medicine, 9*, 1188–1203.

Helgeson, V. (2011). Survivor centrality among breast cancer survivors: Implications for well being. *Psycho-Oncology, 20*(5), 517–524.

Hodge, D. (2004). Spirituality and people with mental illness: Developing spiritual competency in assessment and intervention. *Families in Society, 85*(1), 348–358.

Hodge, D. R., & Bushfield, S. Y. (2006). Developing spiritual competence in practice. *Journal of Ethnic and Cultural Diversity in Social Work, 15*(3/4), 101–127.

Jo, S., Brazil, K., Lohfeld, L, & Willison, K. (2007). Caregiveing at the end of life: Perspectives from spousal caregivers and care recipients. *Palliative & Supportive Care, 5*(1), 11–17.

Jones, B. A., Dailey, A., & Calvocoressi, L. (2005). Inadequate follow-up of abnormal screening mammograms: Findings from the race differences in screening mammography process study. *Cancer Causes & Control, 16*, 809–821.

Kerr, M. E., & Bowen, M. (1988). *Family evaluation*. New York, NY: W.W. Norton.

Kim, Y., Carver, C., Spillers, R., Love-Ghaffari, M., & Kaw, C.-K. (2012). Dyadic effects of fear of recurrence on the quality of life of cancer survivors and their caregivers. *Quality of Life Research*, *21*(3), 515–525.
Kim, Y., Carver, C. S., Spillers, R. L., Crammer, C., & Zhou, E. S. (2011). Individual and dyadic relations between spiritual well-being and quality of life among cancer survivors and their spousal caregivers. *Psycho-Oncology*, *20*(7), 62–770.
Kim, Y., Kashy, D. A., Spillers, R. L., & Eans, T. V. (2010). Needs assessment of family caregivers of cancer survivors: Three cohorts comparison. *Psycho-Oncology*, *19*(6), p573–p582.
Koenig, H. G., & Bussing, A. (2010). The Duke University Religion Index (DUREL): A five-item measure for use in epidemiological studies. *Religion*, *2010*(I), 78–85.
Lambert, S., Jones, B., Girgis, A., & Lecathelinais, C. (2012). Distressed partners and caregivers do not recover easily: Adjustment trajectories among partners an caregivers of cancer survivors. *Annals of Behavioral Medicine*, *44*(2), 225–235.
Maxwell, T., & Aldredge-Clanton, J. (1994). Survivor guilt in cancer patients: A pastoral perspective. *Journal of Pastoral Care*, *48*(1), 25–31.
Miller, W. R., & Thoreson, C. E. (2003). Spirituality, religion, and health: An emerging research field. *American Psychologist*, *58*(1), 24–35.
Mollica, M., & Nemeth, L. (2015). Transition from patient to survivor in African American breast cancer survivors. *Cancer Nursing*, *38*(1), 16–22.
Montesinos, F., & Luciano, C. (2016). Acceptance of relapse fears in breast cancer patients: Effects of an ACT-based abridged intervention. *Psicooncologia*, *13*(1), 7–21.
Morris, B., Leporte, S., Wilson, B., Lieberman, M., Dunn, J., & Chambers, S. (2014). *Journal of Cancer Survivorship*, *8*(3), 427–436.
Morrow, E. M., & Nicholson, C. (2016). Carer engagement in the hospital care of older people: An integrative literature review. *International Journal of Older People*, *11*(4), 298–314. Also in Wiley Editing Services & Wiley Online Library, https://dol.org/10.1111/opn.12117.
Natarajan, L., Minya Pu, B. A., Parker, C. A., Thomson, B. J., Caan, S. W., Flatt, L. M., … Wael, K. L. (2009). Time-varying effects of prognostic factors associated with disease-free survival in breast cancer. *American Journal of Epidemiology*, *169*(12), 1463–1470.
National Alliance for Family Caregiving. (2007). *Resources for caregivers*. New York, NY: Metropolitan Life Insurance Company. Retrieved March 7, 2007, from http:ww.caregiving.org/pubs/brochures
National Cancer Center Institute (2014). *Cancer screening overview for health professionals*. Bethesda, MD: National Institute of Health.
Naus, M., Ishler, M., Parrott, C., & Kovacs, S. (2009). Cancer survivor adaptation. *Journal of Clinical Psychology*, *65*(12), 1350–1359.
Olivetto, I., Gomi, A., & Bancej, C. (2002). Influence of delay to diagnosis on prognostic indicators of screen-detected breast carcinoma. *Cancer*, *94*, 2143–2150.
Park, C., Zlateva, I., & Blank, T. (2009). Self identity after cancer: "Survivor", "victim", "patient", and "person with cancer". *Journal of General Internal Medicine*, *24*(Supp 2), S430–S435.
Peek, M. E., & Han, J. H. (2004). Disparities in screening mammography: Current status, interventions and implications. *Journal of General Internal Medicine*, *19*(2), 184–194.
Rabow, M. W., Hauser, J. M., & Adams, J. (2004). Supporting family caregivers at the end of life: "They don't know what they don't know". *Journal of the American Medical Association*, *291*(4), 483–491.
Rosedale, M. (2009). Survivor loneliness of women following breast cancer. *Oncology Nursing Forum*, *36*(2), 175–183.
Skalla, K. A., Smith, E. M. L., Li, Z., & Gates, C. (2013). Multidimensional needs of caregivers for patients with cancer. *Clinical Journal of Oncology Nursing*, *17*(5), 500–506.
Sklenarova, H., Krumpelmann, A., & Haun, M. W. (2015). When do we need to care about the caregiver? *Cancer*, *121*(9), p1513–p1519.

Spiegel, D., Sephton, S. F., Terr, A. I., & Stites, D. P. (1998). Effects of psychosocial treatment in prolonging cancer survival may be mediated by neuroimmune pathways. *Neuroimmunomodulation, 840*, 674–686.

Taplin, S. H., Clauser, S., Rodgers, A., Breslau, E., & Rayson, D. (2010). Interfaces across the cancer continuum offer opportunities to improve the process of care. *Journal of the National Cancer Institute, 2010*, 104–110.

Teno, J. M., Clarridge, B. R., Casey, V., Welch, L. C., & Wetle, T. (2004). Family perspectives, on end of life care at the last place of care. *JAMA, 291*(1), 88–93.

Van Hook, M., Hugen, B., & Aguilar, M. A. (Eds.). (2001). *Spirituality within religious traditions in social work practice*. Pacific Grove, CA: Books/Cole.

Zeilani, R., & Seymour, J. E. (2012). Muslim women's narratives about body change and care during critical illness: A qualitative study. *Journal of Nursing Scholarship, 44*(1), 99–107.

Chapter 13
Experiencing Cancer Services: A Personal Story of Survival

Jack Phelan

This chapter will provide a personal account of an individual's experience following the diagnosis of cancer and his story of the challenges and barriers that he faced during his illness. Following this, a brief description of several interventions and suggestions is described in an attempt to inform oncology healthcare providers to better serve their patients.

The Initial Reaction

My awareness that I might have cancer started with a sore throat. I gradually had trouble swallowing, even opening my mouth fully. Initially I was treated for a throat infection, and then a lump formed, and it became more serious. I was snowbirding in Arizona at the time and was advised to return to Canada for treatment. Within a few days of medical visits back home, I knew I had cancer.

I am from a family of six children, and my younger sister had been diagnosed with Bartholin gland cancer just 12 months before this. I had lost a brother-in-law to bone cancer in August, and my brother, the youngest, had been diagnosed quite unexpectedly with brain cancer 1 month prior to me. My response to all this was to be embarrassed that I was adding to everyone else's distress with another cancer diagnosis. I had been a regular support for my sister, who had both lost her husband after a very difficult 2-year ordeal and simultaneously begun her own journey of survival. My brother and his wife had recently visited us in Arizona, and he was in great health and looking forward to retiring in 6 months at the age of 60 years. They were totally devastated by his diagnosis, which was quite negative. I believed that my own distress was less significant or important than either of my siblings, and

J. Phelan (✉)
Mac Ewan University, Edmonton, AB, Canada
e-mail: phelanj@macewan.ca

T. R. Fitzpatrick (ed.), *Quality of Life Among Cancer Survivors*,
https://doi.org/10.1007/978-3-319-75223-5_13

I was reluctant to even discuss my own cancer problem. My wife and our three adult sons were more worried than I was, and they became frustrated with my denials and rationalizations. Yet I was convinced that the best way forward was to refuse to take the cancer issue too fatalistically.

From the outset, I thought of my throat cancer as less serious and important compared to the rest of the family. I also never believed that I would not survive this, even though I strongly believe that I will eventually die of cancer, just not yet. So my attitude from the outset was to downplay my cancer, since to me it was comparatively not that big a deal. My story about what had happened to me was powerfully influenced by the more tragic events experienced by my siblings. This awareness of the narrative I was creating and the external forces co-constructing my story will be the framework of this chapter.

I will be referencing the work of Jerome Bruner (1990), a psychology faculty member at New York University, and his work on "meaning-making." Most of the references will be from the book *Acts of Meaning*, published in 1990 by Harvard University Press. My argument is that the meaning intended or assumed to have been delivered by healthcare professionals is often not the actual message received by the patient, not because of language or terminology issues but because of more personal, situational factors. I will be describing my own experience as a cancer patient to illustrate this. The narrative which I have constructed about having cancer is strongly influenced by the experience of having my predictable journey through life disrupted by this major event, which Bruner would describe as a turning point. "And at critical junctures, 'turning points' emerged, again culturally recognizable, produced almost invariably by an access of new consciousness aroused by victory or defeat, by betrayal of trust, and so on" (Bruner, 1990, p. 121).

The Treatment Begins

I had an appointment with my regular GP, who immediately sent me to a lab for a biopsy. The technicians there were very friendly, almost joking as they proceeded to take fluid out of the bump in my neck. I ended up with some bruising, and the results were forwarded to my GP who then sent me to a neck surgeon. He informed me that I did indeed have cancer, but not the type indicated by the lab technicians. He then took a biopsy which was much less intrusive. This was my first experience of poor practice and the less-than-precise world of cancer services, and my skepticism started to grow. This surgeon eventually became the only medical professional that I truly trusted, and I will detail the reasons later.

I was scheduled for a dental checkup and a further, more intrusive biopsy which entailed getting minor surgery in the hospital and then sent to the cancer clinic for an appointment with my oncologist. The throat surgeon met with me after the biopsy and informed me that there were two options going forward: I could undergo a very intrusive surgery, where my jaw would be broken, a piece of my tongue and throat would be removed, a skin graft from my arm would be used as a replacement, and possibly a tracheotomy would be required before having chemotherapy and radiation, or I could forgo that operation and just have the chemotherapy and radiation. He stated that his experience after 15 years of practice is that in my specific case, the success rate would be 85% with the operation and 80% without the operation. I chose to go forward without the throat operation, and he said he would include this in his report.

The Cancer Clinic

I spent 2 days in orientation at the cancer hospital prior to meeting the oncologist. This process solidified my new status as a cancer patient, which was an intimidating and disheartening experience, in spite of the cheerfulness of the nurses and technicians. This included being fitted for a radiation mask, dietary advice, blood tests, and counseling services. I was informed that I must get a feeding tube inserted in my abdomen prior to beginning radiation, since I will have trouble swallowing during my treatment. I was weighed and measured and asked about medication history.

My interview with the oncologist was frustrating. He entered the room holding my chart, which he had not yet read, and had to stop and read my name in the middle of saying hello. He wondered aloud if I actually had cancer to his nurse, who assured him that I did. He then read the chart and stated that I still needed to have the operation on my neck before proceeding. I stated that I chose to just have the chemotherapy and radiation without the operation. He said that this was not possible, since the operation was required. I insisted that this was not what I wanted and that the surgeon had agreed with this decision. He went back to reading the surgeon's report and stated, very unhappily, that he would check with the surgeon, but he did not agree with this.

The Feeding Tube

The nurse practitioner at the cancer clinic told me that I would be required to have a feeding tube inserted before I received radiation and chemotherapy. She said that some people managed to not need this, but it would be too complicated and painful to insert it after radiation had commenced, so everyone got it done. I tried to refuse this, but I was told that it was mandatory. I was scheduled to have it done a week before the radiation and chemo began. The hospital ward for this surgery was busy, and I was inserted at the end of the day, apparently to the unpleasant surprise of the surgeon. He expressed his frustration to the nurse within my earshot, and later the nurses openly discussed their own unhappiness with being asked to work too hard, while I was lying on a gurney in the same area. I asked the surgeon if it would be problematic to do this procedure later in my treatment if needed, since I was told that it was much more complicated to have it done mid-treatment. He said it was not more complicated, and he did not know why I was told that it was. The day following the surgery I had an appointment at the Cancer Clinic to loosen the valve on my abdomen, but the nurse who was supposed to do it was not available, and the nurse who was filling in did not know how to do it, so a nurse was called off the floor to help.

Within a few days, I had an infection at the surgical site and was prescribed an antibiotic, which upset my stomach just as the chemo and radiation were commencing. After a week, during which the infection got worse and my stomach distress was high, I was told that the lab results on my infection indicated that I needed a different type of antibiotic, which then started another 10-day cycle of stomach upset, compounded by the radiation distress. When I saw my oncologist that week and he asked me how I was coping, I described this misdiagnosis and wrong medication. He chastised me, saying it was not the wrong medication but that it was correctly prescribed for what they thought was wrong. I got angry at this but kept quiet. This feeding tube was a major annoyance throughout my treatment, and I believe that I did not need it. It was removed a month after my radiation treatments ended, and it was the beginning of my recovery and belief that I was no longer a patient.

Conflicting Narratives

My experience as a cancer patient, which I have validated in discussions with other patients, is a profound loss of control over one's life and a deep experience of vulnerability and helplessness. In my case, it was counterbalanced by an unwillingness to submit and place my fate in the hands of people whom I had little reason to trust. I did not believe that they had my best interests at heart, even though I did know that they had basic competence and ethics, because I often saw them caring more about themselves and less about me. The story that propelled me included the fact that I was unique, not a statistic or nameless patient, and that I expected excellent performance from each medical professional. The story that I experienced too often from the medical professionals was that they were busy, were stressed, and saw me as a typical case, requiring the usual handling. The literature handed out and the verbal orientations made it very clear that each patient is unique and will receive the exact treatment that is right for them. Yet everyone seemed to get the same number of radiation appointments, for the same duration of time and the same chemotherapy approach.

Each time I saw the oncologist, I was weighed on a scale that had a chart next to it converting kilograms to pounds. On at least three occasions, these handwritten charts disagreed in the conversion equations, and I was offhandedly told by a nurse that this was a well-known but unimportant glitch. It did not increase my confidence in the treatment. I believe that the meaning intended by the medical staff did not match the meaning that I constructed, and this was both unimportant and unnoticed by most of them.

The Throat Surgeon

This man was the most powerful influence on me during this time because he was the only one that I truly believed in and trusted. I will describe the factors which created the connection that supported me throughout the 15 months of my treatment. Some of it will sound trite, but it was very significant. Each appointment with him only lasted 15–20 min, no longer or shorter than other interactions with the team of medical professionals, yet he understood my narrative, and our meaning-making process was focused on me, not him.

He did some typical good bedside manner things, asked me about myself, etc., but he actually listened and shared some of himself, which surprised me. Then he offered me choices, not just diagnostic information, and told me that I was responsible for deciding my own treatment (to a point). He stated that he could see that surgery may not be the best option for me and laughed as he said it may seem unusual for a surgeon to offer that opinion. The simple message I received from him, which struck a deep chord, was that what I needed was more important than what he needed. This was the message that I needed to hear from everyone on the treatment team, but he was the only one that I heard it from.

Another small but powerful thing he did was call me the same day that he did my biopsy, at 8 o'clock at night (he did the biopsy in surgery at 8 am), to tell me the results, since he knew I would be worried. I am still impacted by this simple kindness.

Nine months after my radiation treatments were finished, my oncologist recommended throat surgery to remove some lymph nodes in my neck. I don't know if I would have agreed to this, since I had no faith in the oncologist and there was no immediate crisis, but this surgeon met with me and assured me that it was a useful procedure which he would perform. He asked me to suggest a convenient time based on my schedule (another rare comment), and I had it done. He came to see me in the recovery area at the hospital each day and released me a day early based on my request to leave. The surgery was successful and everything has been fine since. He somehow joined my narrative at each juncture, and I never felt vulnerable or helpless with him.

The Oncologist

In contrast, I have never felt comfortable or even understood by this doctor. He somehow managed to sound insincere even as he was saying hello. I believe that he saw me as a nameless, faceless patient who required the usual, typical treatment, based on my general diagnosis. He would have forced me to undergo a very intrusive surgery prior to radiation and chemotherapy, which I resisted. Six months after the radiation was completed, he examined me in a follow-up visit and read my chart, where he commented "It was a good thing that we agreed not to do that surgery," taking at least some credit for the decision.

Two weeks into the radiation, I had terrible sores in my mouth and on both sides of my tongue. I asked him about this, and he said that since I have caps on my teeth, the radiation bounces off the gold inlays and injures my gums and tongue. He recommended chewing gum to coat my teeth before radiation appointments. I have a mouth guard which I wore subsequently which alleviated this problem, but I was very annoyed that this issue only arose because I mentioned it. I later had constipation for over 3 weeks and was very worried about how this complication was affecting me. He told me to use over-the-counter laxatives and had me X-rayed. He did not give me any reassurances or advice other than to be sure to let him know when I had a bowel movement. I was later told by a nurse that I only had a 35% blockage of my bowel and was not in trouble. This would have been a helpful information while I was worried.

Finally, and most powerfully, after all the radiation and chemo were completed, I had the body scan procedure to determine if I was now cancer-free. I had the procedure on a Thursday morning and anxiously awaited a phone call with the results. I did not hear on Thursday or Friday and spent a very nervous weekend hoping to hear good news. Monday afternoon I finally called the oncologist's office, and his secretary said that she would ask him to call me. He returned my call on Tuesday and casually remarked, "Oh no, your results are clear, no more cancer." He seemed genuinely surprised that I was nervous about this. I was very relieved but also quite angry that he did not think about how I was being affected.

My wife accompanied me on all of my visits to this doctor, and she often had to remind me of the instructions and follow-up advice which were verbalized by both the oncologist and accompanying nurses, because I was not paying attention to their words, since I was suspicious of the agenda of these people who obviously (to me) cared more about themselves than my health and recovery.

This seeming lack of empathy and concern by the oncologist poisoned all of my interactions with him and his team. His oblivious attitude was even more annoying because I was so anxious about my vulnerable situation. To quote Bruner (1990), "…people's self-esteem and their self-concept changed in sheer reaction to the kinds of people they found themselves among, and changed even more in response to the positive or negative remarks that people made to them" (Bruner, 1990, p. 109).

Nurses and Other Health Professionals

Most of the healthcare professionals whom I encountered seemed competent enough but could have done a much better job. An annoying behavior, which other patients I interviewed also experienced, is that nurses will talk about you to other professionals as if you are not in the room. It gives the message that you are just a case to be discussed, not a real person. Many nurses also seem quite comfortable complaining to each other about some aspects of their job while you are present. The meaning-making that is very loud for me is that their daily annoyances are sometimes more important right now than you are, which is quite negative.

I had a swallowing coach who stood out for me because she worked competently and was clearly concerned with relieving my discomfort, which was very important to me. Again, she was focused on what I needed, at least for the time she spent with me. The ignoring of the egocentric preoccupation of people who are anxious about their own survival creates both mistrust and resentment, which can impede the healing process. I was much more attentive to the instructions and advice of the swallowing coach, because she was someone that I trusted. Bruner (1990) states, "I believe that we shall be able to interpret meanings and meaning-making in a principled manner only in the degree to which we are able to specify the structure and coherence of the larger contexts in which specific meanings are created and transmitted" (Bruner, 1990, p. 64). This seeming lack of awareness and empathy by many healthcare professionals is a real problem that can and should be addressed more forcefully. When one's life is at stake, a person becomes hypervigilant and egocentric, which requires the healthcare personnel to focus more obviously on the neediness of the patient and stop expressing irritation at the difficulties of their own situations.

Chemotherapy

I had my first of three chemotherapy appointments on the first day of my treatment. The doctor who was administering this was very soft-spoken and approachable, which helped to calm me down, since this was a very intimidating procedure. This session, which lasted for over 5 h, really impressed on me the seriousness of my situation and the reality of having a potentially fatal problem. Also, the eventual impact, which I experienced more than a week later, was quite profound. I felt totally overcome by the effects of the chemo and felt it throughout my body. It was the beginning of the downward journey that would not get better for several months. My second appointment occurred 3 weeks later, and I had an even stronger reaction to this one. I subsequently became very disheartened, in spite of being warned to expect this, and wanted to stop getting treatments. I really had to force myself to attend the daily radiation sessions after this point and felt weakened both physically and mentally. Prior to each chemo session, I had to get a blood test to check my white cell count, and my third chemo appointment had to be postponed for a week due to my white cell count being too high. I was really dreading my final chemo session, and when the appointment date arrived, the doctor decided that he would cancel this procedure, since it was not indicated. I was so relieved that I could have kissed him. Again, I had the experience that I was being treated as an individual, not just a run of the mill case.

A Surprising E-Mail

At perhaps the lowest point in my treatment journey, I received an unexpected e-mail from a man I had never met, who is a colleague of a good friend in another city. This man had the same cancer as I did, and he was a few months ahead of me in the treatment process. He encouraged me to not despair and to persevere, with details of his own struggle, which seems trite as I am writing this, but it was extremely powerful in the moment. I still have not met him, but I feel connected to him in a powerful way, and I also feel very grateful to my friend whose thoughtful intervention on my behalf created such a good impact when I really needed it. Again, the meaning that I constructed from these events is the important thing, and I believe that this was the intended message from both of these men. Bruner (1990) would say that "We interpret stories by their verisimilitude, their 'truth likeness', or more accurately, their 'lifelikeness'" (Bruner, 1990, p.61).

Recommendations for Clinical Practice, Patients, and Family Members

Park (2016) states that patients with cancer who undergo various treatments are faced with the effects of these treatments for the rest of their lives. "It is therefore our responsibility to support them in the best way we know how" (Park, 2016, p. 20). Many physicians and healthcare providers in hospital settings have focused on the medical aspect of treatment for cancer patients; however, medicine alone is not enough. Many institutions and cancer centers do not support psychological care in their patient's treatment plans. Ruddy (2016), who is the director of cancer survivorship at Mayo Clinic, states that doctors need to remember patients may be dealing with the effects of treatment for the rest of their lives. At present many of the psychological care plans are funded by private donors; however, future psychological care programming in hospitals should be included in the hospital budget (Park, 2016). At the Jewish General Hospital in Montreal, Quebec, which is funded by private donors, a cancer support program titled the "Hope & Cope Cancer Wellness Centre" is a freestanding center for people and their families in the community who have had cancer where psychological, educational, leisure, and physical activities and supportive services are provided (Fitzpatrick, Edgar, & Holcroft, 2012). In addition, the center provides in-service training for volunteers and other professionals who are providing care to the clients, where there is a strong focus on the psychological needs of the clients.

Parle, Maguire, and Heaven (1997) have developed a training model for healthcare workers, mainly doctors and nurses, to help reduce the psychological problems experienced by cancer patients. They state that poor communication such as distancing strategies and avoidance is all too frequent due mainly to their own anxiety and skill deficit. Their model includes a role that encompasses "knowledge and skill deficits, self-efficacy and outcome expectancy beliefs and perceived support plays in the ability and willingness of health professionals to assess their patients' concerns" (Parle et al., 1997, p. 231). They suggest that brief problem-focused workshops be developed to address communication deficiencies between the cancer patient and the professionals.

People with cancer, their families, and carers have a high prevalence of psychological stress which may be minimized by effective communication and support from their attending healthcare professionals (HCPs). Research suggests communication skills do not reliably improve with experience; therefore, considerable effort is dedicated to courses that may improve communication skills for HCPs involved in cancer care. A variety of communication skills training (CST) courses have been proposed and are in practice. We conducted this review to determine whether CST works and which types of CST, if any, are the most effective.

These studies add further understanding to the plight and concerns patients experience when given a diagnosis of cancer and are faced with the challenge of undergoing chemotherapy and/or other forms of treatment plus the physical and psychological effects of treatment. Patients frequently experience fears and uncertainty as they attempt to communicate their needs and in turn must have faith in their medical and professional caretakers.

From a personal point of view, this author's experience as a cancer survivor has been a process of reconstructing my story of self and fitting my thoughts, beliefs, and self-esteem into categories that were previously uncomfortable. I am also aware of the new story that my wife, children, and friends have about me, which involves me being frailer and more vulnerable, even if I don't feel this way. The medical personnel whom I encountered as I reimagined myself have all impacted my narrative, some in positive and others in negative ways, and this narrative will influence my future interactions with the health system. Relational awareness and empathy are critical components of the interactions between healthcare professionals and patients, and this message must be part of the training and evaluation of effective medical interventions.

References

Bruner, J. (1990). *Acts of meaning*. Cambridge, MA: Harvard University Press.

Fitzpatrick, T. R., Edgar, L., & Holcroft, C. (2012). Assessing the relationship betweenphysical fitness activities, cognitive health and quality of life among older breast cancer survivors. *Journal of Psychosocial Oncology*, *30*, 556–572.

Park, A. (2016, November). Frontiers of medicine: The forgotten side of cancer care. *The View Point, Time*.

Parle, M., Maguire, P., & Heaven, C. (1997). The development of a training model to improve health professionals skills, self-efficacy and outcome expectancies when communicating with cancer patients. *Social Science & Medicine*, *44*, 231–240.

Ruddy, K. (2016, November). In Park, Alice, (2016). Frontiers of medicine: The forgotten side of cancer care. *The View Point, Time.*

Index

T. R. Fitzpatrick (ed.), *Quality of Life Among Cancer Survivors*,
https://doi.org/10.1007/978-3-319-75223-5

D

E

The manufacturer's authorised representative in the EU is Springer Nature Customer Service Centre GmbH, Europaplatz 3, 69115 Heidelberg, Germany. If you have any concerns regarding our products, please contact ProductSafety@springernature.com

Printed and bound by CPI Group (UK) Ltd, Croydon, CR0 4YY
05/10/2026
02228147-0002